ZIP IT UP

STAY FIT, STAY FOCUSED, STAY FABULOUS

AKASH JAISWAL

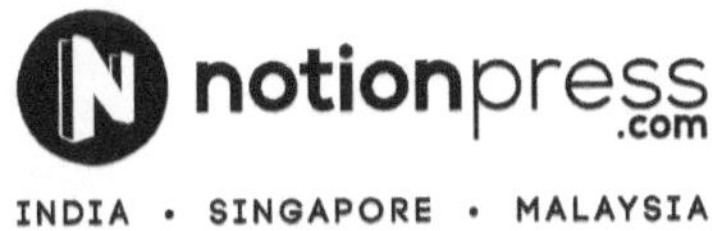

DISCLAIMER

Alright, let's get this out of the way like the broccoli on your plate, important, slightly boring, but totally worth it.

This book is a big ol' mix of health-related stuff you've probably seen floating around, only here, I've tried to make it easier, friendlier, and maybe even fun to read. I've read a ton of research papers (yes, the real kind with scary graphs and tiny fonts) and boiled it all down into something that makes sense. That said, this book reflects only about **10%** of what actually helped me live better. The rest? Life, mistakes, sweat, and stubbornness.

So here's the deal:

Use this book as a **guide**, not gospel. Don't follow everything blindly like a zombie chasing a protein shake. If you have a dietician, trainer, or wellness guru, great! Take this book, wave it in their face, and have smarter conversations. You'll understand your own journey better, and maybe even impress them (no promises though).

All names mentioned are made up or used casually, if they sound familiar, it's purely a coincidence and not me taking a dig at your neighbor. This content doesn't aim to hurt or offend anyone, be it a person, community, race, or even that guy at the gym who never reracks his weights.

Bottom line: The more we know **why** we do what we do, the longer it sticks. And hopefully, with a smile.

DEDICATION

To the Almighty,

I am merely a means of delivering this information. This book would never have seen the light of day had life not shaped me through its lessons and had I not been blessed with proper schooling and guidance. I thank the Almighty for walking with me every step of the way, for whispering hope in moments of despair, and for constantly showing me the path forward.

To my late grandfather,

You were my first cheerleader. I still remember the joy on your face when I handed you my first book. You kept it by your side as if it were a treasure, and that memory still warms my heart. Your belief in me still echoes through everything I do.

To my grandmother,

Your silent strength and unwavering faith have always been my anchor. Thank you for your endless blessings and warm prayers that carry me forward even when the world feels heavy.

To my father and mother,

You are the roots of everything I am. Your sacrifices, support, and love have shaped not just my path, but my soul. Thank you for allowing me to dream freely and to fall, rise, and grow without fear.

To my sister,

Thank you for always being in my corner. Your quiet encouragement and fierce love push me to become better every day.

This book is as much yours as it is mine.

CONTENTS

Stay Fit

Stay Focused

Stay Fabulous

PREFACE

If I could sit face-to-face with my 15-year-old self today, he would probably be speechless. Not because I've suddenly become a superstar or anything like that. But because back then, that boy didn't believe he *could*. He thought being shy, overweight, nervous on stage, and painfully mediocre was the final verdict on his life. That version of me used to question everything, from his abilities to his worth.

Why would anyone listen to me? Why can't I be fit? Why am I not smart enough? These thoughts weren't just occasional, they were everyday companions.

But here's what I would say to that boy now: **"You made it, my man."**

And most importantly, **thank you for not giving up.** Because through all that self-doubt, one thing never wavered: my stubborn refusal to quit. I didn't always know the path, but I always believed there *was* one. And so, I zipped up my hoodie, zipped up my doubts, and just showed up, day after day. I started eating cleaner. I picked up books instead of excuses. I began talking to strangers, learning from their journeys, stepping onto stages, embracing the discomfort, and lifting both weights and my self-confidence along the way. I researched like a nerd, trained like a monk, and failed like a warrior, only to rise again, stronger.

And now? I've written two books, built a healthy lifestyle, and finally, gathered all those little lessons into one powerful, human, and practical guide, **ZIP IT UP: Stay Fit, Stay Focused, Stay Fabulous.**

This isn't just a book. It's your toolkit. Your emotional GPS. Your fitness manual. Your mental reset button. Whether you're that 15-year-old version of me, or someone standing at the edge of change, you'll find your path here. It's not about being perfect. It's about *starting*.

The book is divided into three essential themes:

◈ *Staying Fit*, we dive deep into energy, muscle systems, training techniques, gut health, and why even your best diets sometimes betray you.

◈ *Staying Focused*, we talk about habits, behavior change, the power of intentions, your mind-body connection, and even the ancient Indian wisdom of Ayurveda.

◈ *Staying Fabulous*, because what's the point of progress if you don't *feel* fabulous doing it? Here, we cover body confidence, fashion, aging muscles, product labels, and taking up life's challenges head-on.

From the "Talk Test" to know your cardio threshold to decoding food labels, from understanding why your resolutions fail to embracing your unique style, **this is the book I wish I had when I was lost, stuck, or simply uninspired.** So I wrote it. For you. For the version of you who's about to give up. For the version of you who's just getting started. And for the future version of you who'll say, "Damn, I'm glad I read that."

So, flip the page, and let's start this journey together. Just one promise, when things get hard, you know what to do.

Zip it up... and go get it.

GET MOST OUT OF THE BOOK

"I could never find one book that covered everything about health, nutrition, and the real-life struggles we go through. So I wrote this one."

Simple as that.

You see, I didn't write this to sound smart or throw big fancy words around. I wrote it because I believe that if something helps even one person feel healthier, stronger, or more sorted in life, that's worth it.

As one of my favorite quotes goes:

"Our main business is not to see what lies dimly at a distance, but to do what lies clearly at hand."

This book is your everyday companion, your go-to friend, your nudge in the right direction. This book is not a 400-page thesis that you need to finish and then forget. I encourage you to mark important passages, take notes, and underline passages that resonate with you. Go slow. Come back. Flip randomly. Take your time. Even one grain of sand at a time can make a castle.

"अद्य कर्म कुरु यत्नतः"
But here's a better way to put it:
"Do today's work with full effort."

So don't worry if you skipped a workout, ate that samosa, or felt low yesterday. Today is fresh. This book doesn't demand perfection, it invites progress.

You know what's the shortest distance between you and your goal?

Intention.

Not motivation, not resources, just the decision to try.

Let me tell you a story that changed something in me.

Recently, I visited an old age home. And I met a 70-year-old lady struggling with her MacBook. She had gotten locked out and carried this whole deck of hand-written password cards. She had come all the way, driven herself, just to figure it out. Why?

Turns out, she was writing her memoir, a gift for her children. She didn't want her stories, her lessons, or her memories to go to the grave with her. So, she was learning how to type, how to use tech, and how to ask for help. The determination in her eyes was evident. Man, it wasn't old age. It was pure purpose.

She looked at me and said,
"I just want to complete it. I want to zip it up before I go."

And that hit me. That's all we need sometimes, a reason, a drive, a why.
If she can pull through with that kind of fire at 70, what's stopping us?

So, here's how you read this book:
Don't rush. Pick a section that speaks to you.

Pause often.
Reflect.
Breathe.
Highlight. Re-read.

Take small steps.
One task, one meal, one walk, one workout.

Discuss it.
Talk to your doctor, your gym buddy, or your mom.
Share what you learn.

Apply what resonates. Ignore the rest, for now.

Last Thing Before You Flip the Page
Try motivating someone.
Try listening to someone.
Try believing that small efforts make significant changes.

And above all, try having a goal in your mind, not a big, flashy one. Simply aim for a goal that awakens you with a sense of excitement. That's how you win the day.
Now turn the page… And let's **Zip it Up, together.**

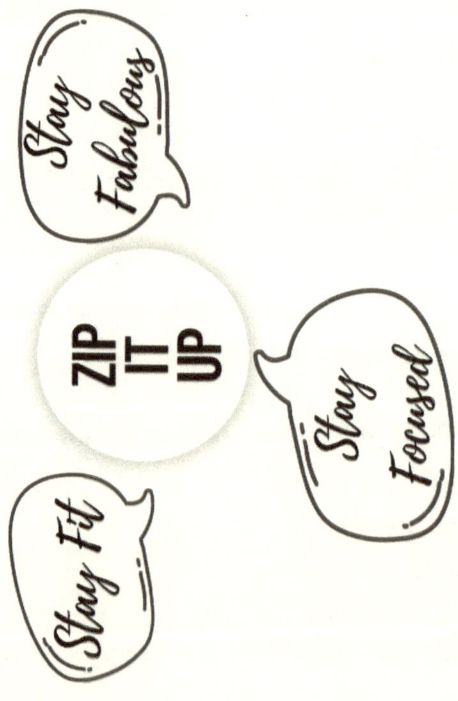

Stay Fabulous
ZIP IT UP
Stay Focused
Stay Fit

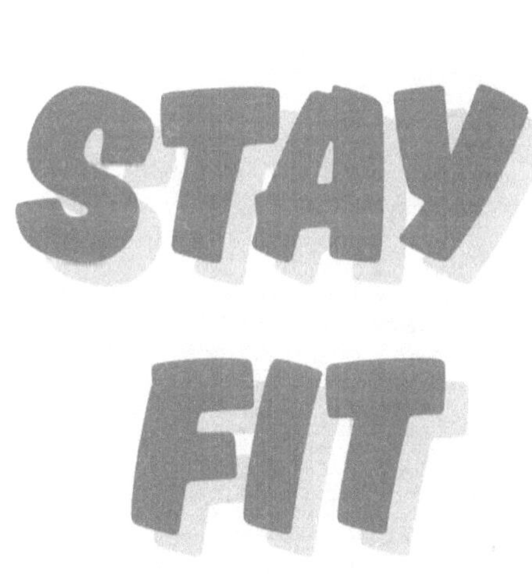

STAY
FIT

DIETING, EXERCISING, AND WHATNOT!!! STILL NOT LOSING WEIGHT?

"Action is the foundational key to all success."

– Pablo Picasso

Have you ever found yourself in this utterly frustrating spot?

You're eating boiled veggies, you're sweating buckets in the gym, aur kya nahi kar rahe ho tum! Still, the needle on the scale doesn't budge.

"Yeh kya bakwaas hai?" You groan, slamming the weighing machine aside.

Well, dost, welcome to the complex and mysterious world of body set weight.

The Body's Secret Thermostat

Our body is not just a simple weighing scale balancing calories consumed and calories burnt. Imagine it more like a stubborn thermostat in your room. Let's say your room's temperature is fixed at 21°C. If you set it down to

0°C, kya hoga bhai? You'll feel chilled to the bone. You bring a heater to warm things up, but as soon as the room gets warmer, the AC kicks in to cool things down. The heater and AC both end up fighting against each other until one of them breaks. This silly fight is precisely what's happening when you diet excessively or overeat.

Science calls this stubbornness **Homeostasis**, your body's way of maintaining a stable internal environment. In simpler terms, your body fiercely defends your "set point weight."

You gain weight?

Metabolism speeds up, appetite goes down, and the body sheds the extra kilos.

Lose weight?

The body slows metabolism, cranks up your hunger hormones (like ghrelin), and conserves energy by dropping your heart rate, body temperature, and blood pressure.

Isliye dieting feels exhausting, you're literally fighting your body's natural thermostat!

The Myth of the Slow Metabolism

You might have thought, "Mera metabolism slow hai, yaar!" But research flips this assumption upside down. Surprisingly, studies show obese individuals actually have higher total energy expenditure than lean ones. For instance, lean people burn around 2400 calories daily, while the obese burn close to

3200 calories, even though they're exercising less! Shocking, right? Your obese body is actually trying hard to lose weight by burning off excess energy.

But phir bhi, you stay obese. Kyun? Because the problem is not the metabolism itself, but your body's set point, it's simply too high!

Let's break it down with a desi example.

Imagine your body's weight thermostat is fixed at 90 kg.

You cut calories and drop to 81 kg.

Initially, you'll celebrate, but soon enough, your body kicks in emergency measures.

Hunger hormones surge, metabolism slows, and you start feeling cold, tired, and hungry all the time.

"Yaar, bas ek samosa kha loon?" Soon, you regain the lost weight.

Classic dieting story, isn't it?

Why Overeating Isn't Actually the Problem

Now here comes the most fascinating twist, overeating is not the primary villain! Eating more doesn't make you fat. Being fat makes you eat more. Overeating is actually a hormonally driven response to increased hunger signals. But what triggers this hormonal imbalance in the first place? The real villain is your high set point weight.

Insulin Resistance, Body's Resistance Game

Let's take another angle: insulin resistance. Imagine insulin as keys and your cells as locks. Normally, ten insulin keys would let twenty glucose molecules into your cells. But if you become insulin-resistant, the keys don't fit properly, and fewer glucose molecules enter your cells. To compensate, your body produces more keys, more insulin, to get glucose inside. High insulin levels become your new normal, creating a vicious cycle.

And guess what? High insulin levels make you store more fat and feel hungrier. Your body's attempt at homeostasis (stability) has now made weight loss even tougher.

The Revolutionary Truth by Dr. Rudolph Leibel

In a landmark study by Dr. Rudolph Leibel (1995), subjects were deliberately overfed and then underfed. When they gained weight, their bodies ramped up metabolism to burn extra calories. When they lost weight, their bodies reduced energy expenditure to regain the lost weight. This clearly demonstrated our body's aggressive defense of the set weight.

Ab samajh mein aaya? Losing weight feels like an endless fight against your own biology because your body tries hard to maintain its preferred weight.

"Toh phir karen kya?"

For that you have to go through the chapters!!!

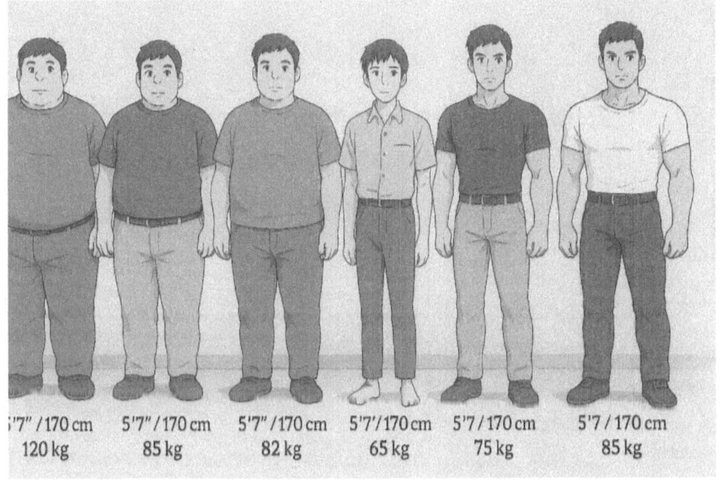

IF YOU ARE NOT SICK, THEN YOU MUST BE HEALTHY!!

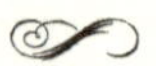

"Health is the greatest gift, contentment the greatest wealth, faithfulness the best relationship."

– Buddha

et's take an example. If a person has lots of stress and muscles are weak and flabby, they probably are not sleeping well. But that one person says, Why should I go to the gym or eat healthy if I am not sick?

What would you think??

Most of us live in the same perception. Does it sound like you?

Then you should keep on reading ahead. Let's consider a hypothetical scenario:

The Wake-Up Call

Aarav Kapoor was the quintessential corporate warrior. Thirty-two years old, living in a high-rise apartment in Bangalore, and scaling the career ladder faster than anyone in his circle. His calendar was a battlefield of back-to-back meetings, client calls, and late-night strategy sessions. The only workouts he knew were typing furiously on his laptop and rushing to catch his next flight.

He wore his "busy" badge with pride.

Sleep? A luxury.

Breakfast? A quick coffee on the go.

Lunch? Who needs it when you can power through with snacks at your desk?

Aarav often laughed off his friends' concerns about his lifestyle, brushing them aside with, "I'm fine! I'm not sick or anything."

But "fine" was a lie. Beneath the surface, Aarav's body was waging a silent rebellion.

One day, his company announced a mandatory full-body health checkup for all employees. Aarav groaned. "Another waste of time," he muttered as he signed up for the earliest slot, hoping to get it over with.

When the test results came back, Aarav's world flipped.

The doctor's words echoed in his head:

"Your cholesterol levels are through the roof. Your liver is showing early signs of fatty liver disease. And you're prediabetic. If you don't make drastic changes now, you're looking at serious health issues within a few years."

Aarav was stunned. *Prediabetic? Fatty liver? But I'm not even 35!*

His mind raced to rationalize it. *I don't feel sick. I work hard, I'm productive, how could this happen?*

That night, Aarav sat alone in his apartment, staring at the report. It felt like a mirror, showing him not just his health but his choices. He thought about the countless skipped meals, sleepless nights, and his body's quiet cries for help, ignored for years.

SOMETHING HAD TO CHANGE....

Well, first, I would tell you some interesting facts. Research published in the Journal of Public Health indicated that approximately 65.4% of participants aged 40 and above in Germany reported regular use of routine health check-ups. The study also found that psychological factors, such as life satisfaction and optimism, were positively associated with the utilization of these check-ups.

The Flawed Binary of Health

Ask all the questions an individual can ask themselves to determine the current health situation:

- Do I wake up feeling refreshed and energetic most days?
- How often do I experience unexplained fatigue or lack of energy?
- Do I experience frequent aches, pains, or discomfort in any part of my body?
- Is my weight within a healthy range for my height and age?

- Am I able to perform physical tasks without undue exhaustion or difficulty?
- Do I experience shortness of breath during routine activities or mild exertion?
- Have I had any significant changes in appetite, weight, or eating habits recently?
- Have I noticed any persistent symptoms such as headaches, dizziness, or digestive issues?
- Do I often feel bloated, lethargic, or hungry after meals?
- Do I have a family history of chronic diseases, and am I taking steps to mitigate risks?

A study from the University of East Anglia found that over 25% of seemingly healthy adults aged 60 and above had undiagnosed heart valve disease. This condition can increase the risk of heart attacks and strokes if left untreated.

So you need to fix your daily routine for your health to catch up with your lifestyle. Some of it you can do is to stop smoking, have a BMI less than 30, and do at least 4 hours of physical activity in a week.

You might have seen lots of commercials saying that you need medications for everything. But your body is not defaulting to get sick. For example, *ZzzQuil* or other sleep aid commercials often depict people tossing and turning, unable to fall asleep, and suggesting that a pill is the solution.

- **Reality Check:** Your body is naturally wired for sleep if given the right conditions, darkness, reduced screen time, and a consistent routine. Sleep aids can disrupt natural sleep cycles if overused.

Don't Wait to Feel Sick to Start Valuing Your Health

Many of us take our health for granted until something goes wrong. We ignore small warning signs, like fatigue, stress, or poor sleep, until they escalate into bigger problems. But why wait for a crisis to act? Your health is your most valuable asset, and the time to invest in it is *now*.

- **Think about this:** If you had a machine worth millions, wouldn't you maintain it regularly to keep it running smoothly? Your body is that machine.
- **Actionable Steps:**
    - Start small: Take a 15-minute walk daily.
    - Replace one unhealthy meal a day with a nutrient-packed option.
    - Schedule that health checkup you've been putting off.

Imagine waking up every day with energy, joy, and the confidence that comes from knowing you're taking care of yourself.

Start your health journey today, not because you're sick, but because you deserve to feel truly alive.

WHAT IS ENERGY? THE HIDDEN FUEL BEHIND EVERY MOVE

"Don't count the days, make the days count."

– Muhammad Ali

Back in school, I used to memorize biology terms like ATP, mitochondria, and glycolysis for marks. I knew all the definitions, diagrams, and cycles. But never in my wildest dreams did I think that one day I'd feel those same processes, not in a lab, but in my body.

From theory to reality, the journey has been wild. I used to be that healthy guy, decent muscles, a little extra fat, vegetarian since birth, living off my mom's legendary recipes and gallons of milk. Life was sorted… until I moved to Kota.

The Rise and Fall Before the Rise Again

In Kota, things got messy. Salty water, messed-up diet, weight gain. Then college came, "Netflix and chill" turned into "Netflix, cheetos, and momos." Studies, late-night bingeing, and zero awareness about health. My body ballooned up, and I didn't even realize it.

But during my master's research, something clicked. Got my stipend, downloaded a calorie tracker, and made a decision. Within 4 months, I dropped serious weight. But man, I looked like a hanger, thin, drained, no strength. That's when I decided to **build** not just a lean body, but a **strong one**.

Weight training began. And over the next 5 years, I stuck to a vegetarian but rigorous diet, consistent workouts, and zero excuses. Eventually, I trained for and competed in a **district-level bodybuilding championship**. Two workouts a day. Clean eating. Cardio. Stretching. No salt. No rice. No water before stage day. That's when the biology I had read came to life.

ATP: The True MVP

Let's talk about the real star, **ATP (Adenosine Triphosphate)**. This tiny molecule is like UPI for your body, quick payment for any action you take. Flex your biceps? ATP. Climb stairs? ATP. Drop your phone and panic-pick it up? Still ATP.

It stores potential energy, and when needed, it **breaks down via hydrolysis**, releasing energy that powers your muscles. It's your internal battery pack, always charging and discharging.

Your Body Has 3 Power Systems: Choose Your Fighter

Depending on what you're doing, your body switches between these energy modes:

1. ATP System (Anaerobic: Sprint Mode)

For those super short, intense bursts, like lifting heavy, sprinting for a rickshaw, or chasing your friend who stole your protein bar.

- No oxygen needed
- Instant power
- Creatine phosphate + stored ATP

2. Anaerobic Glycolysis (Lactic Acid System)

Used when the action goes beyond a few seconds, but still not a marathon. Like doing high-rep sets in the gym.

- Glucose is broken down
- Lactic acid is produced (hello muscle burn!)
- No oxygen used

3. Aerobic System (Endurance Mode)

Now think long walks, cycling, jogging, anything sustainable.

- Oxygen is required
- Uses glucose, fatty acids, even amino acids
- Highly efficient, can go for hours

How Your Body Actually Makes ATP

Here's the simplified science of how your muscles get energy:

- **Glycolysis in Cytoplasm:** 2 ATP made quickly, no oxygen needed

- **Aerobic Metabolism in Mitochondria**: another 2 ATP plus pyruvate for next stage
- **Electron Transport Chain**: The big boss. Makes **34 ATP** from just 1 glucose molecule. Ultimate energy hack.

Muscle Metabolism in Real Life (from Chilling to Championship Mode)

Let me take you through what actually happens inside your muscles in different situations.

1. At Rest

Like when you're watching a cricket match. Muscles are chilling.

- ATP demand is low
- Energy is stored as glycogen and creatine phosphate
- Fatty acids fuel the mitochondria

2. Moderate Activity

Like a regular gym day.

- ATP demand rises
- Oxygen is still enough
- Glucose from glycogen becomes the main fuel
- Fat gets burned if glucose is low

3. Peak Activity

Now picture me 15 days before the championship, training hard, cardio in the evening, posing practice, abs, back-to-back leg days.

- Oxygen can't keep up
- Mitochondria handle only $1/3^{rd}$ of ATP demand
- Glycolysis takes over, causing lactic acid buildup
- Acid levels rise → fatigue hits hard

Muscle Fatigue: When Your Body Says "Bas Karo Bhai"

Even the strongest warriors get tired. In fitness, fatigue comes in different flavors:

- **Endurance fatigue**: When all energy reserves (glycogen, fats) are exhausted
- **Power fatigue**: When lactic acid builds up too fast and muscles stop contracting properly

Trust me, during my 2 a-day sessions, morning heavy lifts, evening 15-minute runs, ab circuits, stretching, cycling, I felt both. But the goal was bigger than the pain.

DOMS: The Trophy You Didn't Know You Earned

Ah, **DOMS (Delayed Onset Muscle Soreness)**. That 24-72-hour soreness after leg day when even sitting on the toilet becomes a challenge.

- Caused by microtears in muscle fibers
- Dull ache, stiffness, sometimes even regret
- But totally normal. And a sign you're growing

Recovery: Where Real Growth Happens

Recovery is your unsung hero.

- Lactic acid is removed through the **Cori Cycle** (it's recycled to glucose in the liver)

- Your body uses **EPOC** (Excess Post-Exercise Oxygen Consumption) to restore ATP
- Muscles rebuild and grow stronger

During prep, I had to make every second count, diet, hydration, sleep, salt control. In the final days:

- Rice stopped 10 days before
- Salt stopped 3 days before
- Water stopped 1 day before
- On the big day, after weigh-in, just 1 katori boiled rice + 1 boiled aloo
- Moov spray + polish for final look and stage heat

Muscle Fiber Types:

- **Fast-twitch (White fibers)**: Power moves. Like chicken breast.
- **Slow-twitch (Red fibers)**: Endurance. Like chicken legs.

Growth & Shrinkage:

- **Hypertrophy**: Training → microdamage → growth
- **Atrophy**: No training → muscle shrinkage.
- After surgery, muscle size can drop drastically in just 1 week

Conditioning: Anaerobic vs. Aerobic

Anaerobic Endurance

- Short bursts (10–20 secs)

- Examples: 50m sprint, pole vault
- Limited by ATP, CP, lactic acid tolerance

Aerobic Endurance

- Long, steady activities (marathons, cycling)
- Needs constant oxygen and fat/carb breakdown
- Best trained through low-intensity, sustained effort

If I hadn't gone through the pain, confusion, discipline, and ultimately joy of transformation, I'd still be that guy who *read* about energy in a textbook. But now, I've lived it.

So whether you're hitting the gym, going for a run, or just starting your fitness journey, remember this:

Your body is capable of magic. ATP is real. Strength is earned. And energy isn't just something you use… **It's something you become.**

Picture this: You wake up late, and suddenly realize you have a 9 AM Zoom call. You jump out of bed, run like Usain Bolt to the bathroom, stretch to grab your towel, and by some miracle, land on your chair just in time. Ever wondered what allowed all that drama to unfold in under 3 minutes? No, it wasn't your willpower. It was your muscles!

Let's take a ride through the most underrated yet most hardworking system in your body, the human muscle system.

What Are Muscles?

Muscles are those stretchy, meaty tissues that help you move, lift, pump blood, smile, breathe, and even digest your butter chicken. They are not just for gym selfies, bhai!

Your body has over **600 muscles,** making up about **40% of your total body weight.** These muscles work either voluntarily (you decide to move them) or involuntarily (they do their job without asking you).

They are broadly classified as:

1. **Skeletal (Striated) Muscles**: Under your control. They help you stand, run, do pushups, and lift heavy bags of rice.
2. **Smooth Muscles**: Found in your stomach, bladder, and blood vessels. They work silently, without any orders.
3. **Cardiac Muscle**: Only in your heart. It beats non-stop. Literally, your most hardworking organ.

Muscles contract and relax. That's their job. Inside them are tiny fibers made of actin and myosin, which slide over each other like kids fighting over a blanket: resulting in movement.

Messages from your brain travel through nerves, instructing muscles to move. This teamwork creates motion, coordination, and that sweet moment when you finally do a perfect burpee.

Let's Explore Muscles Region by Region

Neck Muscles

These help you nod "yes," shake your head "no," and even flex that "what you sayin'?" look. Main players:

- **Sternocleidomastoid**: bends, rotates, and helps in inhaling.
- **Scalene Muscles**: help lift ribs while breathing and rotate the neck.

- **Splenius Capitis and Cervicis**: extend and rotate the neck.
- **Erector Spinae Group**: extends and bends neck sideways.

Back Muscles

Essential for posture and lifting: especially during those PG hostel luggage marathons!

- **Erector Spinae**: extend and bend back.
- **Semispinalis, Multifidus, Rotators**: help in twisting.
- **Quadratus Lumborum**: helps breathing and bends lower spine.
- **Trapezius, Rhomboids, Levator Scapulae**: lift shoulder blades.

Shoulder Muscles

From cricket bowling to throwing chappals, these muscles shine:

- **Deltoid, Pectoralis Major, Biceps, Coracobrachialis**: help in shoulder flexion.
- **Latissimus Dorsi, Teres Major, Triceps**: for extension.
- **Supraspinatus, Infraspinatus, Subscapularis, Teres Minor**: form the rotator cuff.

Arm & Forearm Muscles

From roti flipping to bicep curls:

- **Biceps, Brachialis, Brachioradialis**: forearm flexion.

- **Triceps**: extension.
- **Forearm Flexors/Extensors**: wrist and finger movement.
- **Supinator/Pronator Teres**: rotate the wrist.

Hand Muscles

Small but mighty. Allow us to write, type, play guitar:

- **Thenar and Hypothenar Muscles**: thumb and pinky control.
- **Lumbricals, Interossei**: finger movements.

Abdominal Muscles

More than just for showing off six-pack:

- **Rectus Abdominis**: flexes the trunk.
- **Obliques (Internal/External)**: rotate and flex the trunk.
- **Transversus Abdominis**: compresses abdomen.

Hip & Pelvis

Balance and motion:

- **Iliopsoas, Sartorius, Rectus Femoris**: flex the hip.
- **Glutes (Maximus, Medius, Minimus)**: extend, rotate, stabilize.
- **Adductors, Pectineus, Gracilis**: bring legs inward.

Thigh & Knee

For squats, runs, or catching local trains:

- **Quadriceps (Vastus Group + Rectus Femoris)**: extend the knee.
- **Hamstrings (Biceps Femoris, Semitendinosus, Semimembranosus)**: flex the knee.

Lower Leg & Foot

Helping you walk the talk:

- **Tibialis Anterior, Extensors**: dorsiflexion (lifting foot).
- **Gastrocnemius, Soleus, Plantaris**: plantarflexion (tip-toe).
- **Peroneals**: foot eversion.
- **Flexor/Extensor Hallucis Longus, Digitorum Muscles**: toe movement.
- **Intrinsic Foot Muscles**: stability, arch support.

We humans don't just have big brains; we have smart muscles too! As we evolved, some muscles adapted to support upright walking. Our glutes became posture champions. Our hands evolved for precise tasks, think playing the tabla or threading a needle.

Our **thumbs** got a huge upgrade. Thanks to them, we can do power grips and precision grips: from holding a bat to using a smartphone.

Our face muscles became expressive too. From 'puppy face' to angry boss look: it's all muscles!

Your muscles are your lifelong companions. Treat them right, and they'll carry you far. Exercise them. Feed them. Stretch them. And respect the journey they've made through millions of years of evolution just to let you sit, run, love, live, and dance at baraats!

Zindagi jeeni hai strong, toh muscles banane padenge boss!

ZIP IT, GRIP IT, LIFT IT: MASTERING EXERCISE TECHNIQUES

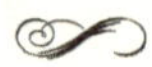

"Champions keep playing until they get it right."

– Billie Jean King

So there I was, first day at the gym. Big mirrors, shiny dumbbells, and a trainer who looked like he could bench press a bike. I walked in confidently… until I picked up the barbell the wrong way and almost folded like a dosa. That's when I realized, **exercise is not just about muscle, it's about method.**

In this chapter, let's uncover the **real science behind doing it right,** whether you're lifting like Rocky or pedaling like a boy. Because **form beats ego,** always.

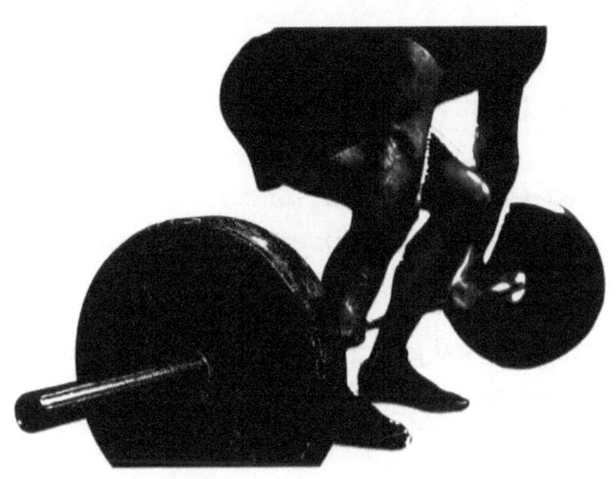

1. Warm-Up: The Unsung Hero

You wouldn't start your car in winter and go full speed in 2 seconds, right? Then why do that to your body?

Start every workout with a **5–15 minute warm-up**, could be a light jog, dynamic stretches, or just dancing to your favorite Bollywood hookstep. It preps your joints, increases blood flow, and mentally gets you in the zone.

And yes, **cool down for 5–15 minutes** too. Let your heart rate settle, stretch those muscles, and sip some paani. Hydration is key, bro, your body loses 2–3.8L water during a workout, so sip like a champ.

2. Form: The Real Flex

Let's break down the basic cues. Whatever exercise you do, free weights, machines, or bodyweight, **your posture, grip, and breathing can make or break your gains**.

Grip Like a Pro:

- **Pronated (palms down)**: used for most pulling motions.
- **Supinated (palms up)**: often for curls.
- **Neutral (handshake grip)**: good for dumbbells or shoulder presses.

And always use a **closed grip** (thumb wrapped) unless you want the bar to say "goodbye" mid-set!

Feet & Body Position:

- For standing lifts: feet slightly wider than hips, heels planted.
- For bench work: use the **5-point contact**: head, shoulders, back, glutes, and both feet grounded.

Breathing Basics:

Inhale when you're going *with* gravity (eccentric) , like lowering the weight. Exhale when you're going *against* gravity (concentric) , like pushing it up. And bhai, please don't hold your breath unless your goal is to recreate a dramatic fainting scene from a daily soap!

3. Machine vs. Free Weights

Machines offer stability, great for beginners or those recovering from injury.

But **free weights**? That's where the real party is.

- They **activate more muscles**, improve balance, and mimic real-life movements.

- Use spotters for heavy lifts and don't hesitate to drop the bar safely if needed (powerlifters do it too, boss).

Use weight belts for heavy squats or deadlifts, but don't become "that guy" who wears it while sipping whey.

4. Cardio Machines

Whether you're burning calories or training for that Goa beach body:

- **Treadmill**: Soft on joints, great control.
- **Elliptical**: Low impact, total body burn.
- **Rowing Machine**: Row, row, row your heart out. Engages both upper and lower body.
- **Stationary Bike**: Low impact, but may tire your legs before lungs.
- **Stair Climber**: Great for glutes, but can stress knees if overdone.

Golden rule: Always breathe easy, and you should be able to hold a conversation.

5. Bodyweight and Nontraditional Training

You don't need fancy equipment. Your body is the best gym.

- **Push-ups, planks, squats**: great for building relative strength and control.
- Want to level up? Try **kettlebells, resistance bands, or tire flips** (yes, Strongman style). These **nontraditional tools** test your stability, coordination, and pure raw strength.

And if you're feeling fancy: **Farmer walks** or **log lifts** give you desi "Khatron Ke Khiladi" vibes.

6. Core & Balance

Abs are made in the kitchen, but **core strength is made in the gym**.

- Include planks, side planks, and standing lifts.
- Use physio balls or unstable surfaces to test your balance.
- Machines isolate, but free weights **activate the core better**.

Remember: **a strong core = injury-free lifting + better posture = confidence**

7. Group Classes & Aerobics: Dance to Fitness

Not everyone loves lifting. Some find their groove in:

- **Low Impact Aerobics**: perfect for beginners, seniors, or pregnant ladies.
- **Step Training, Kickboxing, Aquatic Exercise**: fun, dynamic, full-body workouts.
- **Swimming**: almost full-body, low-impact, and a great life skill too.

Just keep your knees behind your toes, spine straight, and abs slightly tight, **pretend someone's watching you on Bigg Boss**.

Reflecting on my own fitness journey, I recall a time when I was preparing for a local marathon. Despite training rigorously, I neglected proper warm-up routines. On race day, just a few kilometers in, I felt a sharp pain in my calf. That injury set me back weeks. It was a hard lesson on the importance of warming up and listening to one's body.

Another instance was when I attempted heavy deadlifts without focusing on form. Eager to lift heavier, I compromised on technique and ended up straining my lower back. From then on, I prioritized form over ego, ensuring each lift was performed correctly, no matter the weight.

These experiences taught me that in fitness, there's no shortcut. Respecting the basics, warm-up, form, and listening to your body, ensures longevity and progress in the journey.

Exercise is not punishment, it's a celebration of what your body can do. But **doing it right** is what makes it sustainable, injury-free, and truly transformational.

Don't be that guy who lifts heavy with poor form and ends up in physio for 3 months. Be the smart one who trains right, eats well, and **lives like a lion**, quiet strength, loud results.

Let your workouts reflect your story, grit, grace, and a whole lot of sweat.

SELF-ASSESSMENT EXERCISE: EVALUATING YOUR READINESS FOR PHYSICAL ACTIVITY

Before embarking on any new physical activity regimen, it's crucial to assess your current health status to ensure safety and effectiveness. The Physical Activity Readiness Questionnaire (PAR-Q) is a standardized tool designed for this purpose. This exercise will guide you through the PAR-Q to help you determine if you're prepared to increase your physical activity levels or if you should consult a healthcare professional beforehand.

Instructions:

1. **Answer the Following Questions Honestly:**

   - Has your doctor ever informed you that you have a heart condition and recommended only medically supervised physical activity?
   - Do you experience chest pain during physical activity?
   - Have you had chest pain in the past month when not engaged in physical activity?

- o Do you lose balance due to dizziness or have you lost consciousness recently?
- o Do you have any bone or joint problems that could be aggravated by a change in your physical activity?
- o Is your doctor currently prescribing medications for blood pressure or heart conditions?
- o Are you aware of any other reason why you should not engage in physical activity?

2. **Interpret Your Responses:**

- o **If you answered 'NO' to all questions:** You can be reasonably confident that it's safe for you to engage in physical activity. Start slowly and gradually increase the intensity.
- o **If you answered 'YES' to one or more questions:** Consult with your doctor before increasing your physical activity levels. Discuss your PAR-Q responses and follow their advice regarding suitable activities.

3. **Additional Considerations:**

- o If you're feeling unwell due to a temporary illness like a cold or fever, postpone physical activity until you recover.
- o If you're pregnant or suspect you might be, consult your healthcare provider before starting or modifying your physical activity routine.

CREATE YOUR WORKOUT REGIME

"Success is usually the culmination of controlling failure."

– Sylvester Stallone

Let me take you on a little journey, my fitness journey. Imagine a lanky Indian guy, named Akash, whose best workout, once upon a time, was climbing up two flights of stairs, panting as if he'd scaled Everest. Fast forward to today, yes, I'm the same Akash who eventually found his passion in bodybuilding, even bagging a district-level bodybuilding title.

What changed? Everything.

Especially my understanding of how to **CREATE MY WORKOUT REGIME.** But, it wasn't as easy as making Maggi!

Let's dive right in and talk about something every fitness enthusiast must grasp, **THE GENERAL ADAPTATION SYNDROME (GAS).**

Think of your body as an obedient student who reacts predictably to your strict teacher-like commands. When you first hit it with weights, your body enters the **ALARM**

PHASE, sore muscles, fatigue, you name it. But soon, like a jugaadu Indian student, it figures out how to cope. Welcome to the **RESISTANCE PHASE**, where muscles adapt and grow stronger. Ignore your body's signs though, and you risk moving into the **EXHAUSTION PHASE**, which is basically your body shouting, "Bas karo, jaan loge kya?"

Now let's talk about the **FITNESS-FATIGUE PARADIGM**. Have you ever wondered why you're sometimes stronger after a rest day? It's simple: your body recovers (Fatigue decreases) and boom, strength and performance rise (Fitness increases). Here's the catch though, maintaining a balance between your training load and rest is as important as salt in your dal, little less and it's bland, little more and it ruins everything.

Then comes the interesting part, **HYPERTROPHY**. Hypertrophy is the process of muscle growth. Essentially, when you lift weights, tiny tears occur in your muscle fibers. Your body, being the perfectionist it is, repairs and grows these fibers thicker and stronger. This is how we sculpt our dream physique. But muscles don't grow overnight. It's a marathon, not a 100-meter dash. Patience and persistence!

Now, how do you know if your workouts are effective? This is where **TESTING FOR EVALUATION** comes into play. You must periodically assess your progress using certain parameters, strength tests, body composition, aerobic capacity, flexibility, and balance tests. This is your personal reality check. Trust me, numbers don't lie, even when your mirror sometimes does.

Let's shift gears and understand the **7 PROGRAM DESIGN VARIABLES** crucial for building your perfect workout:

1. NEEDS ANALYSIS: Evaluate your goals and needs. Figure out exactly what you want. Remember, clarity is power!

Before anything, you need to understand why you're even lifting that first dumbbell. Whether it's fat loss, muscle gain, or just feeling more confident in your own body, a workout plan without a clear goal is like hitting the road without a map.

Process goals: Walk 10,000 steps daily, stretch after every workout

Performance goals: Increase squat by 10kg in 8 weeks

Outcome goals: Reduce body fat by 5% in 3 months

2. EXERCISE SELECTION: Choose exercises that align with your goals, core exercises like squats and deadlifts for strength, assistance exercises for muscle isolation, and plyometric exercises to boost power and speed. And please, for God's sake, stop doing those fancy moves from Instagram without understanding them properly, safety first!

Strength is the foundation of all movement. Your plan should include:

- **Core Exercises** (Squats, Deadlifts, Bench Press)
- **Assistance Exercises** (Lunges, Dumbbell Rows)
- **Power Moves** (Clean & Jerk, Power Clean)

Aerobic Training: Build Your Engine

Cardio isn't just about fat loss, it's your heart's strength training.

Types of training:

- **LSD (Long Slow Distance):** 60–70% VO2max (Ex: jogging)
- **Tempo:** Threshold training at lactate level
- **Interval Training:** Short bursts, high VO2max
- **HIIT:** Work above 90% VO2max
- **Fartlek:** Desi style "kabhie tez, kabhie dheere" running

3. TRAINING FREQUENCY: Training 3-5 days per week is ideal. More isn't always better. Recovery is when actual muscle building happens. Overtrain, and you're essentially wasting your time. Been there, done that!

4. EXERCISE ORDER: Prioritize compound movements first (think squats, bench presses), followed by isolation exercises (think biceps curls, leg extensions). This ensures maximum efficiency and reduces injury risk.

Keep intensity levels flexible:

- Power: <10 sec, 2–5 reps @ 60–70% 1RM
- Strength: 1–5 reps @ 75–93%
- Hypertrophy: 6–12 reps @ 70–85%
- Endurance: 12+ reps @ <50%

5. TRAINING LOAD AND REPETITIONS: Decide your weights based on your goal, heavy weights with low reps for strength, moderate for hypertrophy, and lighter weights with high reps for endurance. Follow the 2-for-2 rule: if you easily exceed your rep goals in consecutive sessions, increase the weight. Simple maths, right?

Want to move like Virat Kohli between wickets? That's where **speed and agility** drills come in.

- **Rate of Force Development (RFD)**
- **Change-of-direction (COD)**
- **Agility in response to stimuli** (like dodging an opponent)

6. VOLUME: This refers to total workload. For hypertrophy, go for 3-6 sets of 6-12 reps. For strength, stick to 3-5 sets with fewer reps. And yes, more sets don't mean more gains. More smart work, less unnecessary sweat!

7. REST PERIODS: Rest appropriately, 2-5 minutes between sets for strength, 30-90 seconds for hypertrophy, and under 30 seconds for muscular endurance. And I'm not talking about checking Instagram stories during your rests, stay focused!

Speaking of rest, let me briefly touch upon PERIODIZATION, which is just a fancy term for structuring your training throughout the year. Plan your training cycle through Preparatory, Transition, Competitive, and Active Rest periods.

You can't push full throttle all year. Your body needs phases, just like a movie needs plot twists.

Enter **periodization**, the art of cycling through training phases:

1. **Preparatory Period:** Low intensity, high volume to build base fitness
2. **Strength Phase:** Increase weights and reduce reps
3. **Power Phase:** Train for explosiveness
4. **Tapering/Active Rest:** Recover and rebuild

This not only prevents burnout but also ensures peak performance exactly when you need it, be it a competition or your cousin's wedding!

Before I give you the exercise blueprint, I want you to know your body and strength first.

Assess Yourself, The Fitness Baseline

Testing is not just for students. In fitness, it helps you understand your starting line.

Use tests like

- **1RM (One Rep Max):** for strength
- **Yo-Yo Test / 2.4km run:** for endurance
- **T-test / Pro Agility Test:** for agility
- **Push-ups/Sit-ups:** for muscular endurance

Not everyone trains the same. And that's the beauty of personalization.

Kids (6–13): Use light resistance, 1–3 sets of 6–15 reps, focus on form.

Older Adults: Prioritise safety, flexibility, and endurance.

Pregnant Women: Avoid high temperatures, supine positions after the 1st trimester.

Obese Clients: Low-impact, higher frequency. Start with walking, swimming.

Diabetics: Monitor blood sugar pre- and post-exercise

Put It All Together: Your Weekly Blueprint

*** Please check with trained practitioner before following ***

Day	Focus	Key Elements
Monday	Upper Body Strength	Bench Press, Rows, Core
Tuesday	Aerobic + Plyo	LSD Jog + Box Jumps
Wednesday	Lower Body Strength	Squats, Lunges, Calf Raises
Thursday	Mobility + Rest	Yoga, Walking
Friday	HIIT + Core	Sprint Intervals, Planks
Saturday	Group Training	Circuit or CrossFit-style
Sunday	Recovery	Light walk, Massage, Stretch

Workout Like It's Personal

Fitness is not a one-size-fits-all t-shirt from Sarojini. It's your tailored sherwani.

Your regime should reflect *your* life, *your* goals, and *your* struggles.

You don't have to be a gym rat. You just have to be consistent.

And on the days you feel low, remember this line:

"If you can train your mind to show up, your body will follow."

Let this chapter be your *starting point*, your training buddy, your motivational kick. Before I wrap up, let me remind you, everyone is unique. Don't blindly copy Virat Kohli's or Hrithik Roshan's regime, your workout should reflect your individual goals and body's response. Be patient, consistent, and above all, ENJOY the process. Fitness is a lifelong journey, not a quick weekend getaway.

Now, armed with this blueprint, create your regime. Experiment, adapt, evolve. Fitness is not just about looking good in the mirror, it's about feeling strong, confident, and proud. And who knows, maybe someday your story will inspire others, just like mine inspired you!

Get ready to own your journey, let's go, champ!

TALK TEST FOR VENTILATORY THRESHOLD: GAUGING YOUR FITNESS THE EASY WAY!

Imagine this, you're jogging comfortably in your local park, breathing steadily, and suddenly your best friend, Rahul, joins you mid-run and starts pestering you with random questions like, "Yaar, kal ka match dekha kya? Kohli ka shot mast tha!"

At first, you reply with ease, discussing every boundary and wicket enthusiastically. But then, as Rahul increases his pace, you notice your replies getting shorter. Soon, you're struggling to complete even one sentence without gasping for air, finally blurting out, "Abey chup kar na! Meri jaan nikal rahi hai!"

Congratulations, my friend, you just performed a "Talk Test," a brilliant, simple, yet scientifically backed way to check your ventilatory threshold!

Understanding Ventilatory Threshold (VT)

Let's get a little scientific, without making it too heavy. Your ventilatory threshold is the point during exercise when your breathing rate starts to sharply increase, meaning you're switching gears from comfortable aerobic exercise (with sufficient oxygen) to intense anaerobic exercise (where oxygen becomes a luxury!). Basically, your body starts shifting energy sources due to higher intensity, increasing the accumulation of lactate (hello, sore muscles tomorrow!).

The Talk Test is a practical method to pinpoint this threshold without needing fancy lab equipment or expensive fitness watches. Simply put, if you can speak comfortably, you're likely exercising below your ventilatory threshold. If you struggle to say even a short sentence, congrats, you've hit or passed your threshold!

Why Should You Care About the Talk Test?

Researchers have shown how accurate this simple test can be. A study in the Journal of Sports Science & Medicine highlighted that the Talk Test correlates closely with objective measures of ventilatory threshold. Another research published in PubMed (yeah, scientists seriously test everything!) confirms that people who used the Talk Test could effectively maintain optimal intensity without overtraining or injuring themselves.

Here's why I absolutely love this method:

- **It's Free:** Unlike your monthly gym subscription, your voice costs nothing!
- **It's Practical:** You can do it anywhere, on a treadmill, in the park, or even climbing stairs.

- **Self-Regulation:** You naturally adjust your exercise intensity according to your fitness level.
- **Prevents Overtraining:** Keeps you safe by signaling when you're pushing too hard.

How to Conduct the Talk Test Properly:

Follow these easy-peasy steps:

1. **Start Slowly:** Begin your activity at a comfortable pace.
2. **Speak:** Try saying a simple sentence or phrase, like "All is well!" or "Kitne aadmi the?" from Sholay, something short, memorable, and humorous!
3. **Increase Intensity Gradually:** Slowly speed up your activity.
4. **Keep Talking:** At regular intervals, attempt to speak your chosen sentence.
5. **Evaluate:**

   - Easy to speak: You're below threshold.
   - Slightly difficult: Approaching threshold.
   - Struggling or gasping: You've reached or crossed your threshold.

I remember this vividly. My friend Gaurav was preparing for a marathon, determined to prove his fitness. He bought fancy fitness trackers, heart rate monitors, and even downloaded multiple fitness apps. But guess what worked best? The Talk Test!

One day, I joined him for training, and as we ran, I casually asked him about his recent Goa trip. Initially, he described every detail, beaches, parties, seafood, effortlessly. As we picked up the pace, the details started shrinking into mere "Goa mast tha," then finally degraded to desperate gasps of "Paani… please…" That day, Gaurav realized he had unknowingly crossed his threshold, adjusted his pace accordingly, and later credited the Talk Test for optimizing his marathon prep!

Studies suggest that exercising near the ventilatory threshold not only improves cardiovascular health but also significantly enhances endurance. A study published in the National Library of Medicine even found that individuals who regularly performed the Talk Test showed greater improvements in overall fitness compared to those relying solely on heart rate monitors or perceived exertion scales.

The Talk Test isn't just science, it's common sense wrapped in simplicity. For every fitness enthusiast, beginner, or seasoned athlete, this is a handy tool to maintain safe yet effective training intensity. After all, fitness should be enjoyable, not torture!

So next time you lace up your shoes, call a friend, start talking, and train smarter, not harder. Remember, fitness is not just about running faster or lifting heavier, but also about being aware, listening to your body, and having some fun along the way.

EATING ALL RIGHT THINGS STILL STUCK WITH OBESITY

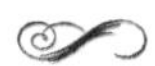

"The last three or four reps is what makes the muscle grow. This area of pain divides the champion from someone else."

– Arnold Schwarzenegger

The Answer You Are Looking For… Is FASTING.

Arrey bhai, tell me honestly, how many times have you started a diet only to give up because of a wedding, festival, or that one friend who always insists on "Bhai, ek bite le le, bas ek"?

Yes, I know you have been struggling to manage your work-life balance, Juggling between **deadlines, chai breaks, midnight Maggi cravings,** and somehow trying to stay fit. And then you start blaming either your **work** or your **personal life** for why you can't follow a strict diet.

But here's a thought, What if you didn't need to follow a strict diet at all?

What if the secret to lasting health, energy, and weight control had nothing to do with counting calories or eating 'perfectly' every few hours?

The answer lies in something much simpler, something deeply rooted in Indian culture, FASTING.

Fasting: Our Desi Wisdom That Science is Just Catching Up To

From your dadi's vrat during Navratri to your Muslim friends observing Roza in Ramadan, to our elders telling us to fast on Mondays or Ekadashi, fasting is something we've always done! But back then, it wasn't just about devotion, it was about **giving the body a break.**

Even the word **BREAKFAST** comes from 'Break-the-Fast,' because traditionally, humans didn't snack all day like we do now.

But today, we are in **full-time feasting mode,**

- Morning: **Chai with biscuits**
- Mid-morning: **Office pantry ka free namkeen**
- Lunch: **Full plate daal-chawal**
- Evening: **Samosa or bhutta (because Mumbai rains or Delhi ki sardi, bro!)**
- Night: **Dinner followed by kheer (because mummy ne banaya hai, toh kaun mana karega?)**

Aur phir, weight loss ka rona.

This constant eating means **our insulin is always high**, making it difficult to burn fat. Studies show that intermittent fasting helps regulate hormones like **insulin, ghrelin (the hunger hormone), and cortisol (the stress hormone).**

For example, intermittent fasting has been shown to **reduce insulin resistance by 20-31%,** significantly lowering the risk of Type 2 diabetes. *(Source: NCBI, 2020)*

"Bhai, Fasting Karna Matlab Bhooka Marna?"

Arrey, not at all! Think about this, The last time you had a **mild fever or flu,** what was the first thing your body did? You lost your appetite. Why? Because your body was prioritizing **healing over digestion.**

This is the body's way of saying, 'Bhai, abhi digestive system ko chhutti de, energy ko kahin aur lagana hai.'

And that's exactly what fasting does, it redirects energy towards healing, fat burning, and mental clarity.

What Happens When You Fast?

Your body goes through different phases:

1. **Feeding (During Meals):** Insulin rises, glucose is stored, and excess energy turns into fat.
2. **Post-Absorptive Phase (6-24 hours):** Insulin drops, glycogen (stored sugar) breaks down for energy.
3. **Gluconeogenesis (24-48 hours):** Liver starts making new glucose from amino acids and glycerol.
4. **Ketosis (1-3 days):** Fat stores break down into ketones, which fuel the brain and body.
5. **Protein Conservation Phase (After 5 days):** Growth hormone rises, **preserving muscle** and lean tissue.

One of the biggest myths is that fasting will make you **lose muscle**. That's **total bakwaas.**

Your body only starts breaking down muscle **when body fat levels drop below 4%,** which is an extreme condition even for bodybuilders!

Fasting actually **preserves** muscle mass because of the increase in human growth hormone (HGH), which helps in fat loss and muscle retention.

"Par Bhai, Fasting Mein Bhookh Lagegi Na?"

Dekho, **bhookh aayegi, par chale jaayegi.** Hunger comes in waves. It's like your annoying landlord calling for rent, just ignore it, and it'll go away for a while.

Common Myths About Fasting, Busted!

- ✗ Fasting will make me weak: Nope! In fact, fasting boosts energy and mental clarity.
- ✗ Brain needs glucose: Partially true, but ketones are an even better energy source.
- ✗ Fasting slows metabolism: No! It actually boosts metabolism by up to 14%.
- ✗ Fasting makes you overeat later: Studies show people do not overeat excessively after fasting.
- ✗ Fasting means nutrient deficiency: If you eat nutrient-dense foods, your body gets everything it needs.

How to Start Fasting: Desi Style

There are multiple ways to do intermittent fasting:

16:8 Method: Fast for 16 hours, eat within an 8-hour window.

24/36-Hour Fast: Full-day fasting, but eat properly when you break it.

Alternate Day Fasting: Eat normally one day, fast the next.

5:2 Diet: Eat normally for 5 days, restrict calories for 2 days.

Time-Restricted Eating: Eat all your meals within a fixed 4-12 hour window.

What to Consume While Fasting (Aur Kya Avoid Karna Hai?)

- ☑ Water: Stay hydrated, bhai! 2-3 liters per day.
- ☑ Lemon Water / Cucumber-Infused Water: Adds taste without breaking the fast.
- ☑ Apple Cider Vinegar (ACV) in water: Helps digestion.
- ☑ Tea (Green, Black, Herbal, Oolong): No sugar!
- ☑ Coffee (Black, No Sugar, No Milk): Can help suppress appetite.
- ☑ Bone Broth / Vegetable Broth: Adds electrolytes.
- ✗ NO Artificial Sweeteners: They trick your body into craving more sugar.
- ✗ NO Juice or Soft Drinks: Even if it says 'sugar-free.'

Breaking a Fast: Don't Attack Food Like a Starved Bhukkad!

Don't overeat immediately, **start with something light** like nuts, soup, or yogurt.

Low magnesium levels can cause muscle cramps, so eat magnesium-rich foods.

Why The Best Diet is No Diet At All

Bhai, dieting is **like an Indian wedding,** too many rules, too many restrictions, and by the end, you're just left confused and frustrated.

Fasting is **simple.** It works **with your body, not against it.**

Diets fail because they're unsustainable. But fasting? **That's just how we were meant to eat.**

So, next time someone says, "Bhai, dieting kar raha hai?", just smile and say, "Nahi bhai, bas **fasting** kar raha hoon!"

Are you ready to take control?

Chalo, let's get started, with FASTING!

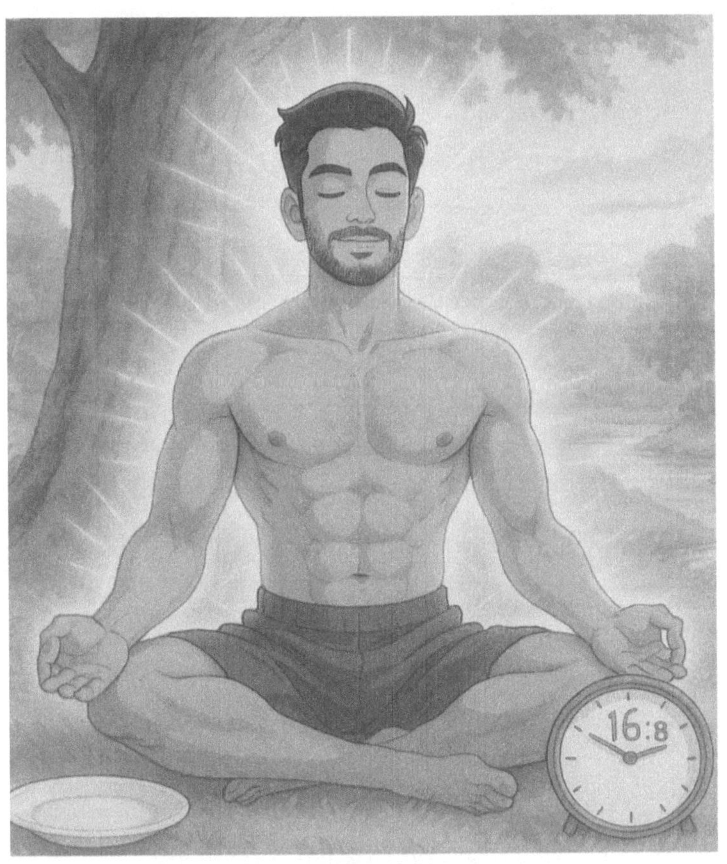
16:8

ZIP UP NUTRITION

"It's not whether you get knocked down; it's whether you get up."

– Vince Lombardi

The FIRST thing we do when we start on fitness journey is to KILL CALORIES

Everyone I met till now is trying to eat less and workout more

I myself did the same

I stopped eating out

I stopped taking in most of the calories

Whether it would be coming from vegetables, junk or fruits

Does that help me??

Initially it helped, and I started to reduce weight

But then I started to get agitated and hormonal changes being to happen

I became lethargic

Also after a while this strict diet stopped giving results

Again I came back to my routine and increase more than that I was reducing

In a meta-analysis of 29 long-term weight loss studies, more than half of the lost weight was regained within two years, and by five years more than 80% of lost weight was regained.

So, how to overcome this issue that I…faced….

Also what happen is that cortisol level increases, which in turn increase blood sugar level and might also increase waist to hip ratio

This can lead to obesity as well.

Instead of focusing solely on restriction, I've learned the importance of a balanced approach, one that includes mindful eating, regular physical activity, and understanding my body's needs.

Let's shift the narrative from dieting to sustainable lifestyle changes!

Every food you eat sends signals. It can turn genes on or off (called **epigenetics**). It shapes your gut bacteria (called **microbiome**). It can even impact your mood, immunity, and mental clarity. So, eat like your future depends on it, because it does. Your Body is a Reflection of Choices. You don't need to follow complicated diets or fancy gym plans. What you need is Real food, Regular meals, Smart hydration and Mindful movement.

When I started my fitness journey, I used to believe that exercise alone could shape my body. I would lift heavy, run fast, sweat buckets, but still, something wasn't clicking. My body didn't reflect the hard work. That's when I realized: **you can't out-train a bad diet**.

What is Healthy Eating, Really?

Healthy eating isn't about eating less. It's about eating right. It's a **balance between fuel and function**, between what your body *needs* and what your *taste buds* want.

A healthy diet includes:

- **Right proportions of macronutrients** (Carbs, Proteins, Fats)
- **Micronutrients** (Vitamins & Minerals)
- **Hydration**
- **Fiber and Phytonutrients**

Think of it like building a house. Macronutrients are your bricks and cement. Micronutrients? They're the electricity, plumbing, and paint, small things, but without them, the house won't function. The Mediterranean diet is considered the gold standard. It's rich in fruits, veggies, whole grains, and healthy fats. But in India, we can recreate it with:

- Dal, sabzi, roti (whole grain), seasonal fruits
- Cold-pressed oils, nuts, and seeds
- Buttermilk, curd, and good hydration

Why Nutrition Matters in Exercise

Exercise is only half the story. Food is the **fuel**. It:

- Powers your workouts
- Reduces injury and illness
- Helps you recover and grow stronger

And no, just protein shakes won't cut it. In our Indian homes, food is love. But when you're working on your body, food also becomes **science**. Our bodies need six essential nutrients to perform, repair, and recover: **carbohydrates, proteins, fats, vitamins, minerals, and water.** Yep, pani bhi nutrient hai!

Carbs & Fats for energy, **Protein** for muscle repair, **Vitamins & Minerals** for metabolism, **Water** as the medium for all reactions

The Basics: Food Is Fuel, Not Just Flavour

1. Carbs: Your Body's Battery Pack

Carbohydrates are not the villain, bro. They're your body's **primary source of energy**, especially when you're pushing yourself in workouts. Stored in your muscles as glycogen, carbs are what help you finish that last set, not faint in it.

Ideal intake: 45-65% of your daily energy

Good sources: Whole grains, rice, oats, fruits, legumes

Pro tip: Choose low-glycemic index carbs, they release energy slowly. Don't binge on sugar-laden snacks and expect six-pack abs.

2. Protein: The Repair Mechanic

You can break your muscles in the gym, but protein repairs and builds them stronger. They're made of **amino acids**, some essential (can't be made by your body), some non-essential (body makes them, chill).

Protein need based on your training:

- Sedentary life: 0.8g/kg body weight
- Moderate exercise: 1.2-1.4g/kg
- Intense training: Up to 2.2g/kg

Sources: Eggs, fish, chicken, dairy, soy, dal-chawal combo for vegetarians.

And yes, **vegans can also build muscle**, if their diet is planned right. Ever heard of rajma-chawal gains?

3. Fats: The Misunderstood Friend

Not all fats are bad. Your body needs fat to absorb **vitamins A, D, E, K** and to make hormones (yes, including testosterone). But choose the right fats!

Good fats: Olive oil, nuts, seeds, avocado, fatty fish

Limit: Trans fats, deep-fried samosas, and packet chips

Let's not ruin our goals over weekend cheat meals turning into cheat weeks.

4. Vitamins & Minerals

These don't give you energy, but they support every function inside your body, from immunity to healing, to making your bones strong. Think of them as the **bolts holding your Ferrari together**.

Best way to get them? Eat the rainbow, different fruits, veggies, whole grains, dairy, and nuts.

5. Hydration

Water is not just for thirst. It's for muscle function, fat burning, digestion, and even brain sharpness. Lose just **2% of your body water** and your performance drops like Sensex after budget day.

Daily need: 8-12 cups (more if you exercise)
Best indicator: Clear urine, like limca, not fanta

Before workout: 400–600 ml (2-3 hours before)
During workout: 200 ml every 15-20 min
After workout: 500–700 ml per 0.5 kg of sweat lost
Hack: Weigh yourself before and after gym. 0.5 kg drop = 500 ml water needed.

For intense workouts or cardio in Indian summers, switch to **isotonic drinks** to replenish electrolytes.

Pre-Workout Nutrition: Don't Run on Empty

Ever tried doing leg day on an empty stomach? Feels like trying to climb Himalayas in chappals.

Eat smart before your workout. Meal should be:

- High in carbs
- Moderate in protein
- Low in fat and fiber
- Packed with fluids

Timing tips:

- Big meal: 4 hours before
- Light snack: 1-2 hours before

    Examples: Banana, smoothie, curd, sandwich, pasta
    Remember: You don't need butter chicken before a run.
    You need power, not petrol pump food.

During Workout: For Long Haulers

If your workout is exhausting and lasts **90+ minutes**, especially cardio or sports matches:

- Take 30-60g of carbs per hour
- Hydrate continuously

    Examples: Sports bar, banana, diluted fruit juice

Post Workout: Recovery Mode ON

The golden window of recovery is **within 2 hours post workout**. This is when your muscles are most hungry, like you after a long day at office.

Your meal should be:

- High in carbs + proteins
- Low in fat
- Packed with vitamins and minerals

Examples:

- Grilled chicken with rice
- Mushroom omelette + toast
- Peanut butter and jelly sandwich

Feed Your Goals, Fuel Your Dreams

What is Healthy Eating, Really?

A balance between fuel and functionb, beítran
Macronutrients, Micronurrients
Fiber and Phyonutrients

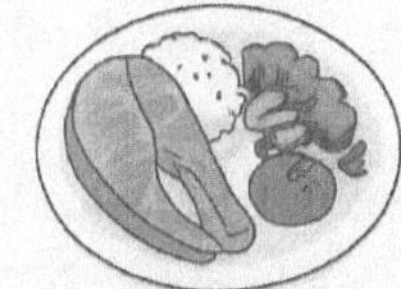

Healthy vs. Unhealthy: The Real Test

Healthy vs, Unhealthy, The Real Test	
Whole foods	Regular meals
Regular meals	Skipping meals
Portion control	Uvere ating
Water, coconu't	Sugary drinks

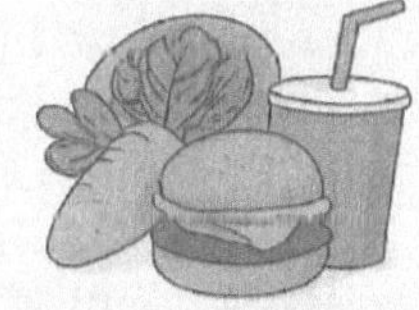

Your 5 Golden Rules for Exercise Nutrition

1 Fat enough **quality prctein**
2 **Stay hydrated** – numbu paní, bíhoí nimbu pani,buttenik
3 **Fuel before workouts**, bananas, oats
4 **Recover smart** – Post-workout meals matter!
5 Don't **skip** meals – Muscles need regular fuel

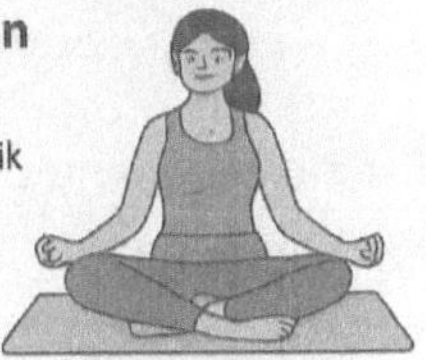

Understand Your Energy Needs

Need or hype.

- Eat enough **quality protein**
- **Stay hydrated** – dal, paneer, egggs, fish
- **Fuel before workouts**. bananas, oats boiledchana
- **Recover smart** – Post-workout meals matter'
- **Don't skip meals**

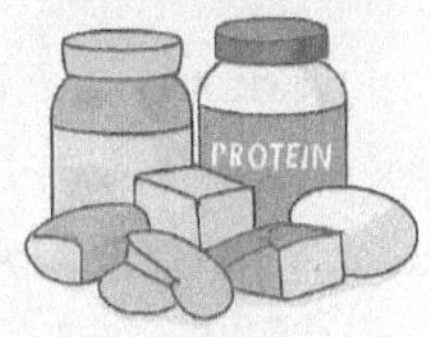

Food is More Than Calories

Every food you eet sends signals — ícthafene-,
impunity, and mental clarity. It can impact.
your body. Feed ít well. And watch ít beconíe

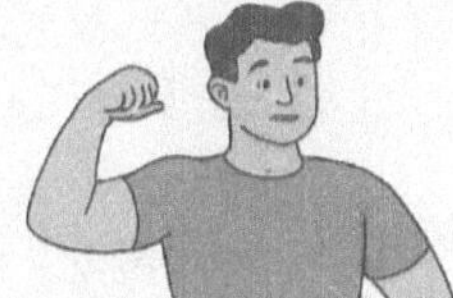

Final Words: Your Body is a Reflection of choices

Real food, regular meals; smart hydration, mindful movement   any et.

Supplements? Not always needed. But if you're not hungry after workouts, a quality protein shake helps. Whey, casein, soy, all have their pros.

The World of Supplements: Real Gains or Marketing Hype?

Let's break it down:

- **Sports foods**: Energy drinks, bars, gels, they're convenient but not your main meal.
- **Ergogenic aids**: Only 5 have solid evidence, Caffeine, Creatine, Nitrate (like beetroot juice), Beta-alanine, and Sodium bicarbonate.
- Creatine is king for strength training. Start with ~0.3g/kg/day for 5–7 days, then maintain with 3–5g/day.
- Beetroot juice boosts stamina, great for joggers and cyclists. 500ml/day does the job.

But no supplement can replace dal-chawal and mumma ke haath ka khana.

Antioxidants? Yes, but not too much. Overdosing on them post-workout can be counterproductive. Trust your plate over pills. Vitamin D and magnesium are two nutrients most Indian fitness freaks lack. Get your levels checked. If your D is low, 2000–5000 IU/day can help.

Popular Diets: Fads or Facts?

Keto Diet

- Super low carb, high fat.
- Can help in fat loss and energy production.

- But watch out for nutrient deficiencies and keto flu (nausea, cramps, sugar cravings).
- May reduce performance in weightlifting or intense workouts.
- Cyclical keto (CKD) works better: 5 days keto + 1-2 days high-carb.

Intermittent Fasting (IF)

- Focuses on when you eat, not just what.
- Time-Restricted Feeding, Alternate Day Fasting, Fasting Mimicking Diet, all versions of IF.
- Can improve sugar control and brain function.
- But not recommended for intense training days.

Low FODMAP Diet

- Best for people with bloating, gas, or gut issues.
- Athletes with digestive discomfort can try this.
- Avoid sports gels and bars with sorbitol/fructose.
- Go for glucose-based products.

Food Allergies and Intolerances: Know Before You Eat. Some people can't digest certain foods. It's not drama, it's real science.

Food allergies are immune reactions (e.g. peanuts, eggs, shellfish) that can be severe. **Food sensitivities** are delayed reactions, can cause brain fog, bloating, fatigue.

Food intolerances (like lactose intolerance) are enzyme issues.

Athletes must read labels. Sports products often contain hidden allergens. (More on reading label at the end)

Listen to your body. Energy crashes? You're under-eating. Always tired? Maybe you're skipping nutrients. Supplements are like *extra marks* in an exam. They help, but only if your base is strong. Multivitamins, protein powders, omega-3s, good if there's a gap. But don't rely on them like magic pills. This chapter isn't just about what to eat, it's about how to think about food. In India, we are blessed with **diverse, nutritious, and affordable options**. Let's stop chasing the Western "keto-shmeto" madness and return to our roots.

KNOW YOUR BODY, FUEL YOUR FIRE

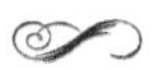

"A year from now you'll wish you had started today."

– Karen Lamb

"Tu apne body ko nahi samjhega, toh kaise banega fit? Pura game wahi se shuru hota hai, bhai."

This chapter is for every desi who has looked in the mirror and thought, *"Yaar, kuch toh karna padega."* But before we jump into crazy diets or buy that fancy gym membership, let's pause and understand the most underrated part of fitness, **knowing your body** and **feeding it right**. You wouldn't drive a car without checking the fuel, right? Toh phir yeh body ka kya?

Let's decode fitness with science, desi style.

You remember ABCD from school? Well, now it's back, but this time, it's about your health:

- **A: Anthropometry:** Measurements of your body, height, weight, waist, hip, BMI. Basically, tape measure aur weighing machine ki yaari.

- **B: Biochemical:** Blood tests and all the lab stuff.
- **C: Clinical:** Doctor ki observations, hair loss? Pale skin? Weak nails? Sab batata hai kuch.
- **D: Dietary:** What you eat daily, roti-sabzi or pizza-burger?

Out of these, the most practical and desi-friendly way to start is anthropometry.

The Magic of Measurements: Anthropometrics. Start with the basics: **height, weight,** and **waist-hip ratio**. Measure these and you'll unlock insights into your body type. Let's break it down:

1. BMI (Body Mass Index)

It's like a report card that tells you if you're underweight, normal, overweight, or obese.

Formula: BMI = Weight (kg) / Height (m^2)

But bhai, BMI has its own tantrums. It doesn't know if you're a muscular guy or just motu. So don't take it too seriously. Ek reference ke liye theek hai.

2. Waist Circumference and WHR

Your tummy matters more than your weight. Yup.

- **Waist-to-hip ratio (WHR)** = Waist ÷ Hip
- **Waist circumference** tells you about risks like diabetes and heart disease.

Too much belly fat? That's a warning bell. Time to cut that midnight maggi.

Bioelectrical Impedance Analysis (BIA). Sounds high-tech? It's that machine in good gyms that tells you your **fat mass, lean mass,** and **water levels**. Kya faayda?

- Know your **intracellular and extracellular water**.
- Understand **BMR (Basal Metabolic Rate),** how many calories your body burns in rest.

How to estimate BMR?

Mifflin – St. Jeor equation

BMR (female): $10*W + 6.25*H - 5*A - 161$

BMR (male): $10*W + 6.25*H - 5*A + 5$

W= weight in kg; H= height in centimeters; A=age

Imagine this: You're just lying down, binge-watching Shark Tank, and still burning calories. That's BMR!

Calculating Ideal Body Weight (IBW)

Not everyone needs to be 6-pack shredded. You need to know your **ideal weight**. There's a formula for that:

For Men:

IBW = (Height in cm – 100) – (Height – 150)/4 + (Age – 20)/4

For Women:

IBW = (Height – 100) – (Height – 150)/2.5 + (Age – 20)/4

Example: For a woman who is 168 cm tall and 33 years old:

= (168–100) – (168–150)/2.5 + (33–20)/4

= 68 – 7.2 + 3.25 = **64 kg**

Types of Body Composition. Sab motapa ek jaisa nahi hota.

- Some people are "skinny fat": dikhenge patle but body fat zyada hota hai.
- Some are muscular but heavy.
- Some retain water.

Understanding your **body composition pattern** is crucial. That's how you'll know whether you need fat loss, muscle gain, or hydration.

Now that you know your structure, let's talk about **fuel**. Your body is like a gadi, needs the right petrol to run smooth.

What Is Energy?

It's the **capacity to do work**. Released by food through metabolism. Carbs, proteins, and fats are our fuel.

1 kcal = 1000 calories = 4184 joules

For daily use, **1 kcal = 1 calorie** (Don't get confused, bro).

- **Total Energy Expenditure (TEE)**

Your energy burn happens in 3 parts:

1. **BMR:** Body at rest, basic survival energy.

2. **TEF (Thermic Effect of Food):** Energy used for digesting food. (Fun fact: protein & spicy food increase it!)

3. **PA (Physical Activity):** Exercise, walking, even standing!

So, total energy needs = **BMR × PA factor × 1.1 (TEF)**

Physical activity (PA) factors for BMR adjustments

Activity factor	Activity level	Explanation
1.2	Sedentary	Little or no exercise. Desk job.
1.375	Lightly active	Little exercise or sports 1-3 days per week
1.55	Moderatly active	Moderate exercise or sports 3-5 days per week
1.725	Very active	Hard exercise or sports 6-7 days per week
1.9 -2.0	Extremely active	Hard daily exercise or sport and physical job

- **Calculating Your Daily Energy Needs**

  Let's take an example.

  A man, 45 years old, 180 cm tall, 85 kg weight, works out 3 times/week:

  BMR = 10×85 + 6.25×180 − 5×45 + 5 = **1755 kcal**

  Energy Needs = 1755 × 1.375 × 1.1 = **~2654 kcal**

One more example:

A 30-year-old woman, 168 cm, 64 kg, strength trains 2x/week + aerobic 2x/week:

Energy needs = **~2351 kcal**

This is to **maintain weight**. For weight loss or gain, you'll adjust from here.

- **Special Case – Overweight Individuals**

  For people with **BMI > 30**, don't use actual body weight directly.
  Use this formula instead:

  Corrected Weight = (Actual weight − IBW) × 0.25 + IBW

Then plug that into BMR and energy calculation.

Body Is Already Burning

You wake up on a lazy Sunday, roll around on your bed, maybe check your phone, and think, "Yaar, aaj toh kuch bhi nahi kiya."

But here's the truth: even when you're doing *nothing*, your body is doing *everything*.

Your heart is beating. Your lungs are expanding. Your brain is processing a million things in the background. Your liver, your kidneys, your muscles, all are working like loyal employees in a factory that never shuts down. This factory is your body. And this body… is already burning.

Activity Over the Ages: From Farming to Facebook

Let's rewind to 1945. The world was recovering from World War II. Food shortages, poverty, and malnutrition were everywhere. So, the United Nations created the Food and Agriculture Organization (FAO) to ensure no one sleeps hungry.

But soon they hit a wall. They didn't know how much food the world actually needed. Why? Because they had no idea how much energy people spent daily. A farmer and a typist don't burn calories the same way, right?

So, scientists came up with a clever metric called **PAL**, **Physical Activity Level**. It tells you how active someone is, by comparing their energy spent in 24 hours to what they'd burn just lying in bed.

Here's the magic:

- A lazy couch potato might have a PAL of 1.4.
- A factory worker, farmer, or construction worker? 2.0.
- Our hunter-gatherer ancestors? About 1.9.

Sounds like they were hyperactive? Guess what, wild animals still burn way more, with PALs of 3.3 and above. Meaning, even our most active ancestors were "lazy" compared to the average street dog in India.

We Were Born to Move… But Chose Chairs

In 1960, about half of all American jobs needed moderate physical work. Today, barely 20% do. We sit, we stare, we scroll. Elevators, cars, remote controls, we've engineered physical effort out of our lives.

On average, people now burn **100 calories less per day** than their grandparents did. That's like skipping a short walk every day. It might not sound like much, but over a year, that adds up to **26,000 calories**, enough to run ten marathons!

And yet, instead of working with our hands to survive, we now have to **choose** to exercise. It's like ordering physical activity from a gym menu just to stay alive. Wild, right?

The Price of Just Being Alive

You think rest is free? Let's break the myth.

A man weighing 82 kg (180 pounds) burns **1,700 calories a day** just sitting in a chair doing nothing. That's your **Resting Metabolic Rate (RMR)**. Your body's basic survival budget.

Even in sleep, your body is working, digesting food, regulating temperature, replacing old cells. Strip that to the bare minimum and you get your **Basal Metabolic Rate (BMR)**, about 10% less than RMR. That's what you burn if you lie in bed all day, fasted, in a cool, dark room, basically, in zombie mode.

Science has now evolved. We don't chase people with oxygen masks anymore. We just check your **pee**. (No kidding!) By analyzing heavy hydrogen and oxygen atoms in your urine, scientists can now calculate your **Total Daily Energy Expenditure (DEE)**. It's creepy science, but cool science.

And guess what? Most of your energy, **63%** , is burnt just to keep your body going. Maintenance. Repair. Defense. No gym needed.

Hadza, Hunger & the Human Machine

Meet the Hadza, one of the last hunter-gatherer tribes in Tanzania. They don't hit the gym. They walk, hunt, build, dig. Yet, after adjusting for body fat, their **metabolism is just like yours.**

Here's the real shocker: humans across the globe, whether they work in New York or in rural Rajasthan, burn roughly **30 calories per kg of fat-free body mass per day**. We are energy-budget machines, regardless of what we do for a living.

Most of our calories, more than 20 trillion across all humans every day, are burnt just to **exist**.

When the Body Goes on Strike. Now, let's stress-test the body.

During World War II, a study called the **Minnesota Starvation Experiment** made 36 men eat almost nothing for 6 months. Just enough to survive. What happened next is what Bollywood might call "shocking and emotional."

They lost 70% of their fat. But that's not the highlight. Their **BMR dropped by 40%**. From 1,590 to 964 calories, the energy needs of a school kid!

They weren't just tired. Their **sex drive vanished**, skin became flaky, they were always cold, and they hardly moved. The body started saving energy like a miser. Muscles shrank. The heart got smaller. Liver and kidney sizes dropped. Even **earwax production reduced!**

Think about it, the body made choices:

- Keep the **brain and liver** alive
- Cut down **muscles and heat**
- Forget about **reproduction or growth**

It was like a country running out of budget, hospitals stay open, but gyms shut down. Pure survival mode.

When you lie down and say, "Bas, aaj kaafi ho gaya," remember this, your body isn't slacking off. It's cleaning, healing, regenerating. Even in silence, there's a symphony inside.

We always think **activity** is costly, but **rest is expensive too**.

So now, here's a mind-bender, should we burn more calories for fitness or conserve them for healing? There's no one answer. It depends on your goal:

- Want to fight infection? Rest.
- Want to lose fat? Move.
- Training for a marathon? Balance both.
- Trying to get pregnant? Prioritize maintenance.

At the end of the day, your body is like a wise accountant, every calorie spent is tracked, evaluated, and optimized. The Bottom Line: Burn Intentionally

The body is always burning. It's not *if*, it's *where*.

You can spend your fire on building strength, healing trauma, chasing dreams, or just surviving.

But here's the truth: **burn with purpose**. Because whether you're building muscle in a Mumbai gym, coding late nights in Bangalore, or just sipping chai after a walk in Lucknow, your body is working hard.

So, respect it. Move it. Feed it. And most importantly, understand it.

Because your body… is already burning.

Fitness starts with self-awareness. The tape measure and calculator can be your best friends, use them wisely.

Apni body ko samjho, fir usse chuno apna fuel. Don't follow trends blindly. What's keto for one may be killer for another. You're not just anyone, *you're YOU*.

And remember, **your fitness is not a punishment. It's a privilege.** Har drop of sweat, every calorie counted, it's not struggle, it's **self-love**. If you're ready, let's move to the next chapter and build a plan that works for you. Not for Bollywood, not for Instagram, **but for the guy or girl in the mirror.**

BMI Classification Table

BMI (kg/m^2)	Classification	Health Risk
Below 18.5	Underweight	Nutritional deficiency, weak immunity
18.5 – 24.9	Normal/Healthy	Low
25.0 – 29.9	Overweight	Increased
30.0 – 34.9	Obesity Class I (Mild)	High
35.0 – 39.9	Obesity Class II (Moderate)	Very High
40.0 and above	Obesity Class III (Severe)	Extremely High

Key Formulas Sidebar

Formula	Expression
BMI	BMI = Weight (kg) / Height (m)^2
Waist-to-Hip Ratio	WHR = Waist (cm) / Hip (cm)
IBW (Men)	IBW = (H - 100) - (H - 150)/4 + (A - 20)/4
IBW (Women)	IBW = (H - 100) - (H - 150)/2.5 + (A - 20)/4
BMR (Men)	BMR = 10*W + 6.25*H - 5*A + 5
BMR (Women)	BMR = 10*W + 6.25*H - 5*A - 161
TDEE	TDEE = BMR * PA Factor * 1.1
Corrected BW	Corrected BW = (Actual - IBW)*0.25 + IBW

THE FORGOTTEN SUPERPOWER INSIDE YOU YOUR GUT

"You dream. You plan. You reach. There will be obstacles. There will be doubters. There will be mistakes. But with hard work, there are no limits."

– Michael Phelps

et me start by telling you a story, not of a king or a warrior, but of a common man. Let's call him Ramesh. A 35-year-old IT guy from Bangalore. On paper, he had it all, a decent job, a good family, and a Netflix subscription. But every day, Ramesh woke up bloated. He felt tired, moody, and low on energy. He'd get random skin breakouts, and his stomach felt like a ticking time bomb, sometimes it was gas, sometimes constipation, sometimes both. And guess what his doctor told him?

"Stress le lo thoda kam, Ramesh ji."

Now here's the twist. It wasn't just stress. The real villain was living inside him: his **gut microbiome**, a dense, invisible world of trillions of microbes that silently control everything from your weight and mood to your skin, energy, and immunity.

Sounds like a sci-fi story, right? But this is science.

Our Modern Gut Is a Mess

Let's face it, our gut is **broken**, thanks to modern life. Over the years, we've bombarded it with antibiotics for every cold, killed the good bacteria with chlorinated water, survived on samosas and Maggi, and said no to dahi and pickles that our dadi used to insist on. This constant abuse leads to a condition called **dysbiosis**, an imbalance in your gut microbes.

And no, this isn't just about your stomach. This is about your *whole body*. Your skin, brain, sleep, hormones, metabolism, everything starts from the gut.

Meet the Silent Villain: SIBO

One of the most common results of a broken gut is **Small Intestinal Bacterial Overgrowth**, or SIBO. It happens when bacteria from the colon decide to party in the small intestine, where they don't belong. Symptoms? Bloating, gas, constipation, brain fog, even anxiety. And the worst part? Most people have no idea this is happening inside them.

Bad Bacteria, Bad Life

Certain harmful microbes like **E. coli, Klebsiella, and Pseudomonas** can cause inflammation, increase insulin resistance (hello, diabetes!), make your skin dull, and even disturb your brain chemistry. Ever wondered why you're constantly craving sugar or feeling irritated? Maybe it's not your fault. Maybe it's your microbes.

The Gut-Brain Love Story

Yes, your **gut and brain are BFFs**. Gut microbes produce neurotransmitters like **serotonin, dopamine, and GABA**. Mess up your gut, and you mess up your mind. That's why people with poor gut health often feel anxious, depressed, or mentally foggy.

So when your mom said, "Sab pet ka problem hai,", she wasn't wrong.

Good Bacteria = Superpowers

On the flip side, certain good bacteria can be your personal health army. They:

- Control hunger and cravings
- Produce happiness chemicals
- Fight inflammation
- Keep your skin glowing
- Slow down aging

You don't need a spa. You need a **super gut**.

The Magic of L. Reuteri Yogurt

Here comes the hero of this chapter, **Lactobacillus reuteri**. This humble bacteria, when turned into homemade yogurt, has been shown to:

- Increase **oxytocin** (the love hormone)
- Reduce appetite
- Boost muscle and skin regeneration

- Elevate your mood
- Make you biologically younger

Yes, seriously.

Dr. William Davis, in his book *Super Gut*, swears by it. He recommends fermenting it for 36 hours with a warm, steady temperature and adding prebiotic fibers to feed the bacteria. No, this is not your regular store yogurt. This is next-level biohacking.

Ramesh's Transformation: The 4-Week Protocol

Coming back to Ramesh, he didn't give up. He followed the **Super Gut 4-week protocol**, and what happened next will shock you more than a plot twist in a South Indian movie.

Week 1: Gut Reset

He ditched sugar, wheat, processed foods, and soft drinks. Started on basic probiotics. And stopped feeding the bad bacteria with junk.

Week 2: Kill the Villains

He introduced natural antimicrobials like **garlic extract, oregano oil**, and **berberine** to kill harmful microbes.

Week 3: Rebuild

He brought in the good guys, fermented foods, prebiotic fibers like **inulin,** and **L. reuteri yogurt**. Bone broth and glutamine helped heal his gut lining.

Week 4: Stabilize

Now that the bad guys were gone and the good ones were flourishing, he focused on lifestyle, better sleep, more movement, managing stress. His energy returned. His belly flattened. His skin glowed.

Tests and Tracking

For those who love data (hello, engineers), there are breath tests for SIBO and stool tests like **Viome** to analyze your microbiome. But even without fancy tests, your body will give signs, clear skin, better mood, lighter digestion, and mental clarity.

Lifestyle Shifts That Matter

- **Sleep**: 7-8 hours minimum. Your gut heals at night.
- **Stress**: Chronic tension ruins your gut flora.
- **Exercise**: A simple 30-minute walk daily increases gut diversity.
- **Avoid**: Artificial sweeteners, painkillers (NSAIDs), and yes, tap water loaded with chlorine.

Probiotic Power Players

Some key strains to look out for:

- **Lactobacillus reuteri**: Skin, love, and longevity
- **Bacillus coagulans**: Digestion buddy
- **Bifidobacterium infantis**: For mood and IBS
- **Akkermansia muciniphila**: For leanness and metabolic health

Immunity, Childhood, and Beyond

Did you know that **70-80% of your immune system** lives in your gut? C-section babies, formula-fed infants, and even adults raised without fermented foods tend to have weaker immunity. But it's never too late to rebuild.

You Are Not Old, Just Inflamed

Aging is not just about grey hair and wrinkles, it's about internal inflammation. And a **super gut can literally reverse signs of aging**. That means you can be 40, but feel and function like 30. No fountain of youth needed, just the right microbes.

Still getting those late-night sugar cravings? It's not your willpower. It's the bad microbes demanding their feed. Once you fix your gut, those cravings vanish like the last slice of pizza at a college party.

So, whether you're a Ramesh, a Ritu, or someone stuck in the daily Indian grind, bloated, tired, anxious, your answer might not lie in another coffee or pill. It lies in your gut. Heal it, and your body becomes your best friend again.

In the end, it's simple: **If your gut is happy, your life is happy.**

And remember, your dadi's achaar wasn't just tasty, it was a medicinal masterpiece.

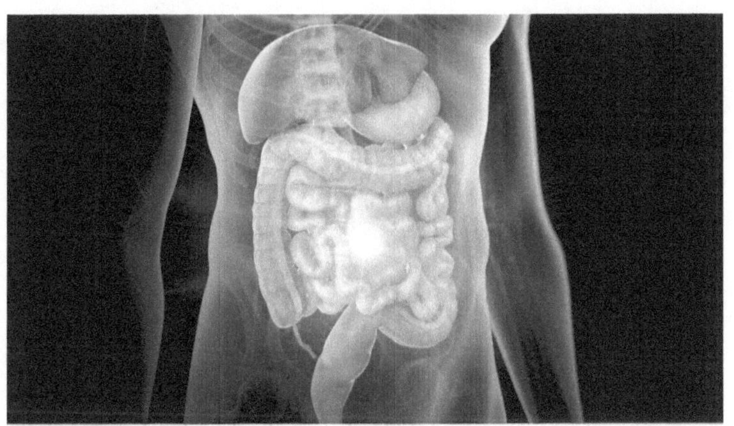

STAY FOCUSED

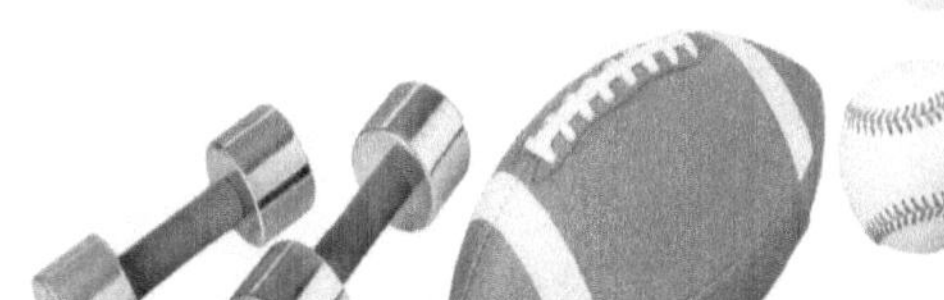

92% OF NEW YEAR S
RESOLUTIONS FAIL.....
THE 1% RULE

"You don't rise to the level of your goals. You fall to the level of your systems."

– James Clear

study by the University of Scranton revealed that most people abandon their goals because they focus on results rather than identity. Similarly, the **Framingham Heart Study** found that if your friends gain weight, you're **57% more likely** to gain pounds too. Habits are contagious, whether good or bad.

When we start on a new habit, we need to check in with these questions:

Is it appealing? Do I want to do it?

Is it achievable? Can I actually do it?

Is it easily activated? Is there a prompt that reminds me to do it?

The aroma of cutting chai filled the air as Amit, Raj, and Sameer sat at a small tea stall in Bangalore. Amid the hustle and bustle of the city, they found themselves discussing something that had been on Amit's mind lately, habits.

"Bro, I was reading this book *Atomic Habits* by James Clear, and it blew my mind!" Amit exclaimed, taking a sip of his chai. "He says that improving just 1% every day can lead to massive results over time."

Raj raised an eyebrow. "1%? That sounds like nothing! How can such a tiny change even matter?"

Sameer leaned forward, intrigued. "That's what I thought too! But think about it, if you improve by just 1% every day, you'll be 37 times better in a year. There's actual math behind it. It's like compound interest, but for your personal growth."

"Exactly!" Amit nodded. "Toyota used this principle in their Kaizen philosophy, continuous improvement. Small, consistent changes made them one of the biggest car companies in the world."

This idea of *tiny but consistent* improvements was life-changing, and they were about to dig deeper.

Why Small Habits Matter More Than Big Goals

"But don't we all set goals anyway? Like, 'I'll lose 10 kg' or 'I'll go to the gym every day'?" Raj asked.

"That's the problem!" Sameer said. "Goals alone don't work. People focus on outcomes instead of identities. Instead of saying, 'I want to lose weight,' say, 'I am a fit person.' Every action then reinforces that identity."

Amit added, "There's a study by the University of Scranton that found *92% of New Year's resolutions fail*. Why? Because people focus on results instead of building an identity. If you want to be a writer, don't just aim to write a book. Say, 'I am a writer,' and start writing every day."

The Habit Loop: Cue, Craving, Response, Reward

"Okay, that makes sense. But how do we actually build good habits?" Raj asked.

"There's a simple formula," Sameer said. "It's called the *Habit Loop*, Cue, Craving, Response, Reward."

- **Cue**: Something triggers the habit (e.g., seeing running shoes makes you think of jogging).
- **Craving**: You feel the urge (e.g., imagining how fresh you'll feel after a run).
- **Response**: You take action (e.g., going for a 10-minute run).
- **Reward**: You get satisfaction (e.g., endorphins make you feel good).

"MIT researchers found that habits are stored in the *basal ganglia* of our brain," Amit added. "That's why forming a habit takes time, our brain needs to wire the new loop."

Make Good Habits Easy, Bad Habits Hard

"Bro, it's so hard to break bad habits. I keep doom-scrolling on Instagram and wasting hours!" Raj complained.

"That's because bad habits are easy and rewarding," Sameer said. "The trick is to reverse the loop. If you want to reduce phone usage, make it invisible, keep your phone in another room. If you want to wake up early, keep your alarm clock away from your bed."

Amit nodded. "BJ Fogg, a behavioral scientist, found that *habit stacking* works wonders. If you already brush your teeth every morning, stack a new habit on top, like doing five push-ups right after."

The Two-Minute Rule: Start Small, Stay Consistent

"But what if I don't feel motivated? Some days, I just don't feel like doing anything," Raj admitted.

"Motivation is overrated," Sameer said. "Instead, focus on the *Two-Minute Rule*. If you want to start a new habit, make it so easy that it takes less than two minutes."

"Like if you want to start reading, don't say, 'I'll read for one hour.' Just say, 'I'll read one page.' Once you start, you'll naturally do more," Amit added. "Newton's First Law, an object in motion stays in motion."

Your Environment and Social Circle Shape Your Habits

"But bro, my friends always order junk food, so I end up eating badly too," Raj admitted.

"That's because *environment shapes habits*," Sameer explained. "It's easier to change your environment than rely on willpower. If you want to eat healthy, keep fruits on the table and junk food out of sight."

Amit chimed in, "A famous *Framingham Heart Study* found that *if your friends gain weight, you are 57% more likely to gain pounds too.* The same applies to positive habits. Surround yourself with the right people."

Breaking Bad Habits: The Inversion of the Habit Loop

"So if I want to quit junk food, should I just stop buying it?" Raj asked.

"Exactly!" Sameer said. "To break a bad habit, invert the habit loop:

- **Make it Invisible**: Keep junk food out of your home.
- **Make it Unattractive**: Watch documentaries on how junk food harms health.
- **Make it Difficult**: Don't keep cash for impulse buys.
- **Make it Unrewarding**: Track your spending on junk food and see how much money you waste."

"A *University of Copenhagen* study found that making bad habits harder to access helps people quit them," Amit added.

Overcoming Immediate Gratification

"Our brain is wired for *temporal discounting*," Sameer explained. "We value immediate rewards over future benefits. That's why junk food, scrolling Instagram, or skipping workouts feels easy."

"But we can bridge the gap!" Amit said. "*Temptation bundling* works, pair something you *want* with something you *should* do. Like, 'I'll only watch Netflix while walking on the treadmill.'"

Optimize Your Surroundings to Change Habits

"Your surroundings play a huge role," Amit continued. "For example, never go grocery shopping on an empty stomach, you'll end up buying junk. And if you want to move more, take the stairs instead of the elevator."

Sameer added, "Your *social network* matters too. If your best friend works out regularly, *your chances of being active triple.* If they eat healthy, *you're five times more likely to eat healthy.*"

The 1% Journey Begins Now

Raj shook his head, laughing. "Damn, I never thought habits worked like this! We always focus on big changes, but it's really about small improvements every day."

"Exactly! *Atomic Habits* isn't just about productivity, it's a science-backed way to change your life, one small habit at a time," Sameer said.

Amit lifted his chai. "So, let's start our 1% journey today. No more excuses!"

And with that, the three friends made a pact, to build better habits, one tiny step at a time.

"If you can't do everything, do one thing. But *do it daily.* That's how life shifts."

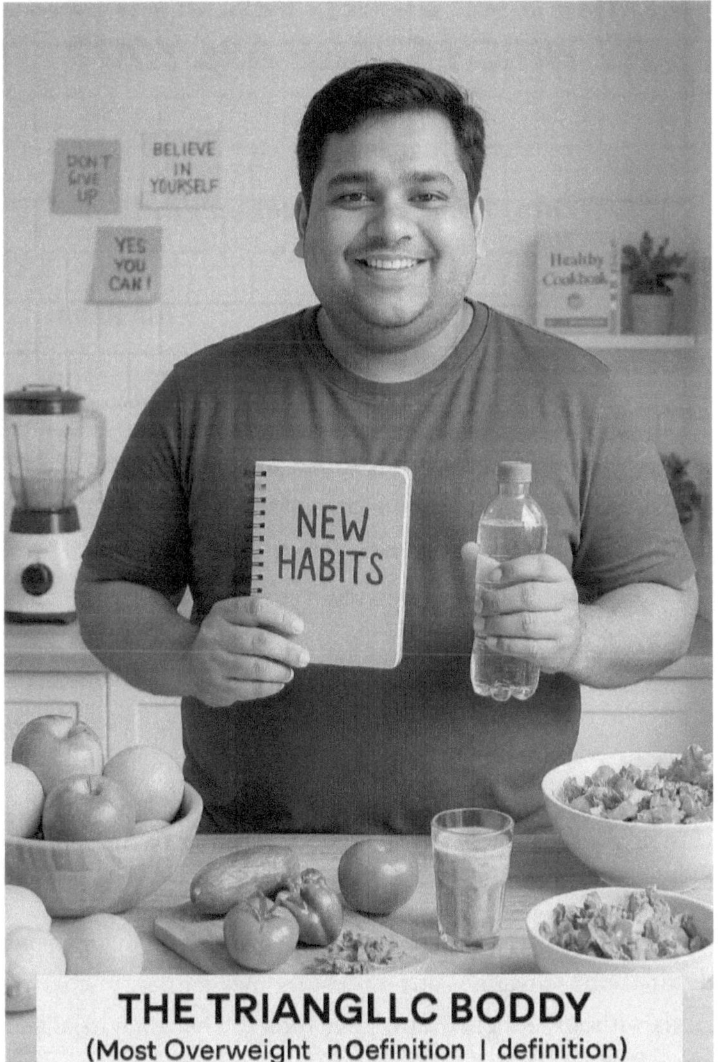

DON'T GIVE UP
BELIEVE IN YOURSELF
YES YOU CAN!
Healthy Cookbook
NEW HABITS
THE TRIANGLLC BODDY
(Most Overweight nOefinition | definition)

STAGES OF BEHAVIOR CHANGE: AT WHICH STAGE ARE YOU?

"Take care of your body. It's the only place you have to live."

– Jim Rohn

I know you feel stuck when it comes to achieving your fitness goals. You start with enthusiasm, but somewhere along the way, life gets in the way, motivation fades, and before you know it, you're back to square one.

Sounds familiar? You're not alone.

The good news is that changing your behavior is not a mystical process. It's not about waking up one day and suddenly becoming a fitness freak. No, it's a journey, a series of steps, like climbing a staircase. Each step gets you closer to the top, but first, you need to figure out where exactly you stand right now.

Would you ever go on a road trip without knowing your destination? Imagine our ancestors navigating uncharted lands without Google Maps. They took the hard way, trial and error. But we live in the 21st century, where knowledge is at our fingertips, yet we still insist on struggling instead of leveraging what's already discovered.

So let's cut to the chase.

If you want to succeed in transforming your health and fitness, there are three crucial things you need to understand:

1. **Readiness for change,** Do you have the resources and knowledge necessary to make a lasting change?
2. **Barriers to change,** What's holding you back from making the shift?
3. **Relapse likelihood,** What could cause you to slip back into old habits?

Once you understand these, you can navigate through the six stages of behavior change, as defined by James O. Prochaska and Carlo C. DiClemente in their Transtheoretical Model (TTM). These stages are: **Precontemplation, Contemplation, Preparation, Action, Maintenance, and Relapse.**

Let's break them down.

Stage 1: Precontemplation: "Nothing's wrong with me!"

This is the phase of **denial and ignorance**. People in this stage don't recognize that they have a problem.

Let me tell you a familiar story. A guy, let's call him Rohan, was slim and active all through his college years. He played cricket, cycled everywhere, and barely had a belly. Then, he landed a corporate job. Days became a cycle of sitting at a desk for 10 hours, eating junk food, weekend parties, and endless scrolling on Instagram. Slowly, he started gaining weight.

But in his mind, Rohan was still the same fit guy from college. "Oh, I can lose this weight in just a couple of months; I just need to stop eating rice," he told himself. Months passed, but he did nothing.

That's **precontemplation**, where you don't realize the seriousness of your situation. To move forward, you need to **rethink your behavior, assess risks, and analyze how your current lifestyle is affecting your long-term health**.

Stage 2: Contemplation: "Maybe I should do something about it"

At this stage, people become aware of the potential benefits of making a change, but they also focus on the challenges that come with it. There's a constant back-and-forth between wanting to change and staying comfortable. You know you need to start working out or eating better, but every time you think about it, excuses like "I don't have time" or "I'll start next Monday" creep in. Maybe you've even Googled "best diet for weight loss" while munching on a samosa. To move forward, you need to weigh the pros and cons of your current habits and recognize the barriers that are stopping you. The more clarity you have about why you need to change, the easier it becomes to take the next step.

Stage 3: Preparation: "Alright, let's make a plan"

This is the point where you start experimenting with small changes. Maybe you buy new workout clothes, start looking up diet plans, or even sign up for a gym membership. You haven't fully committed yet, but you're warming up to the idea of change. You might even download a fitness app, only to ignore its notifications for a week. The key to moving forward here is to set clear goals and create an actionable plan. Write down why you want to change and how you're going to do it. Having a roadmap will make the journey easier and keep you accountable. Just don't be that person who buys an expensive protein powder before even starting push-ups!

Stage 4: Action: "Let's do this!"

This is the phase where you finally take real steps towards your goal. You've stopped just thinking about it and have started putting in the work. Maybe you've begun exercising regularly, eating healthier, or following a structured plan. You wake up at 6 AM, put on your workout clothes, and finally hit the gym instead of just hitting snooze. This is where consistency matters. To stay on track, reward yourself for small achievements, whether it's losing a kilo or sticking to your diet for a week. Also, don't hesitate to seek social support, having an accountability partner or joining a community can make the process easier and more enjoyable. Find that gym bro or "workout wali dost" who will drag you to the gym when you feel lazy.

Stage 5: Maintenance: "I got this!"

Now that you've developed good habits, the challenge is to sustain them. Many people lose motivation here because the excitement of starting something new fades away. The real test is when you go on a vacation or have back-to-back weddings to attend. Temptations will be everywhere, jalebis, biryanis, and buffets that seem impossible to resist. You must develop coping strategies to ensure your progress doesn't go to waste. Keep tracking your progress, set long-term goals, and remind yourself why you started in the first place. Most importantly, keep rewarding yourself for sticking to your new routine, acknowledge how far you've come. But hey, an occasional gulab jamun won't kill your progress if you're consistent otherwise!

Stage 6: Relapse: "Oh no, I messed up!"

Relapse is a common part of any change process. One bad week doesn't mean you've failed. You might skip workouts, binge on unhealthy food, or fall back into old habits. Maybe you convinced yourself that "thoda zyada kha liya toh kya ho gaya," and the next thing you know, you're back to old patterns. The key is not to dwell on it but to learn from it. Identify what triggered the relapse and recognize the barriers that tripped you up. Reaffirm your goal and commit again, because progress isn't about perfection, it's about persistence. Remember, even Sachin Tendulkar got out on a duck sometimes, but he still went on to score centuries. So get back on track!

Where Are You Right Now?

Now that you understand these stages, ask yourself: **At which stage are you?**

Are you still in denial? Are you thinking about change? Planning? Taking action? Are you struggling to maintain your progress?

No matter where you are, **the key is to keep moving forward.** Fitness isn't about achieving perfection overnight. It's about continuous improvement, one step at a time.

So, don't just sit there contemplating. **Identify your stage and take the next step today!**

FACES FIERCE INTENTIONS

"You are what you do, not what you say you'll do."

– Carl Jung

It was another Sunday afternoon when I found myself glued to yet another fitness guru video on YouTube. I recalled my initial days of confusion, scrolling through videos by legends like Guru Mann, BeerBiceps, and Sahil Khan, hoping to decode the secrets of fitness. Suddenly, I remembered Sahil Khan's epic line, **"Fitness is a lifestyle, not a sprint."** It felt personal, just like he was talking directly to me.

Curiously, one term stood out repeatedly, **'low-fad diet.'** Intrigued, I asked myself, "What's this new fancy word?" Turns out, it's all about cutting refined carbs, your biscuits, cakes, white bread. These comfort foods stimulate our brain's reward system, becoming addictive faster than binge-watching my favorite web series.

Initially, I'd doubt every diet tip. I mean, mice studies? Seriously?

"We are human beings, not lab rats. Trust human studies only!"

That point stuck with me ever since.

Our bodies crave balance, maintaining a delicate state called **Homeostasis**.

Hormones, the messengers of our bodies, play a significant role here. Imagine hormones like delivery agents, efficiently handing messages to targeted cells. Insulin, for instance, guides glucose into cells, similar to your Zomato guy handing over your pizza order, quickly and effectively.

Eating refined carbs spikes your blood sugar quicker than Rohit Sharma's boundaries. According to a 2018 study published in Diabetes Care, refined carbohydrates can spike blood sugar levels dramatically within just 30 minutes of consumption. This rapid rise releases insulin, pushing sugar into cells. Excess carbs get stored as glycogen, akin to mom packing extra laddoos after festivals, handy but limited.

Once glycogen storage maxes out, additional sugar turns to fat, a scientific term called **De Novo Lipogenesis**. Fancy name, same old fat.

Hours later, sugar levels drop, and the liver reverses glycogen storage, turning it back into glucose. Every night, this happens unless you're caught raiding the fridge at midnight (been there!). During extended fasts, your body cleverly converts fat back into glucose, called **Gluconeogenesis**.

Think of insulin as your body's gatekeeper, storing sugar and fat when food is plenty and burning it when fasting. But here's the tricky bit: excess calories convert into visceral fat (around organs), subcutaneous fat (under your skin), or even liver fat.

I vividly remember someone humorously explaining this: **"I can make you fat. Anyone can! Just prescribe prednisone, a synthetic cortisol drug, and you'll balloon faster than roadside pani puri."** Prednisone, used for inflammatory diseases, consistently triggers weight gain by elevating insulin.

Cortisol, known as the stress hormone, prepares your body for threats. Imagine our ancestors escaping tigers, cortisol provided instant energy. Today, we don't face tigers, only bosses, relationships, EMIs, and traffic. Long-term psychological stress (like constantly checking notifications) keeps cortisol and glucose high.

Numerous studies back cortisol's sneaky role in obesity. A landmark study in 1998 demonstrated that volunteers given cortisol showed insulin spikes dramatically, up to 36% above baseline. Chronic cortisol due to stress or lack of sleep (yes, those late-night Netflix binges count!) directly increases insulin resistance and obesity. Even mild cortisol elevations widen your waistline.

Remember Guru Mann discussing Cushing's disease? Excess cortisol leads to inevitable weight gain, despite diet or exercise. A study published in Clinical Endocrinology showed that 97% of Cushing's patients experienced abdominal obesity regardless of their lifestyle.

"Lower stress, lose weight?" Absolutely. Conditions with low cortisol, like Addison's disease, consistently lead to drastic weight loss.

Stress without calories can indeed make you fat. However, binge-watching Netflix or Instagram scrolling isn't stress relief, it's active management through mindfulness meditation, yoga, or regular exercise. Studies conducted by Harvard Health demonstrated that mindfulness practices effectively reduce cortisol and visceral fat.

Sleep is another hidden culprit. In 1910, people averaged about nine hours of sleep per night; today, many barely get six. Research published in the American Journal of Epidemiology showed sleeping less than seven hours increases obesity risk by over 50%. Even one sleepless night spikes cortisol significantly, reducing insulin sensitivity. Persistent sleep deprivation accelerates diabetes and fat storage.

So finally, what's the solution?

Simply ditch refined carbs, actively manage stress, meditate, unplug from devices, and prioritize sleep. As BeerBiceps wisely says, **"Fitness starts with small, sustainable lifestyle changes."** Perhaps these fitness gurus weren't just selling another fad, they genuinely knew the fierce intentions behind lasting health. With these intentions, reclaiming our health becomes possible, one practical step at a time.

THE MIND-BODY CONNECTION: UNLOCKING YOUR INNER STRENGTH

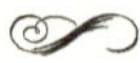

"You miss 100% of the shots you don't take."

– Wayne Gretzky

Mind-body practices like acupuncture, meditation, and mindful exercises have strong neurobiological foundations, explaining how they positively influence critical brain functions.

Scientific research confirms that consistent engagement in mind-body exercises such as Tai Chi, Qigong, and Hatha Yoga effectively improves conditions like hypertension, insulin resistance, chronic pain, cardiovascular issues, anxiety, and depression. These activities provide significant enhancements in balance, strength, flexibility, relaxation, and mental calmness. Additionally, because mind-body exercises are typically low-intensity, easily adaptable, and require minimal equipment, they can be conveniently incorporated into daily routines, making them highly beneficial for many individuals.

Kya boss, kabhi socha hai ki why you feel lighter after chanting Om or doing simple breathing exercises?

No, it's not some magical voodoo; it's pure science, Neurobiology to be exact! Apne hi brain mein setting hai that explains why these ancient practices like meditation, yoga, acupuncture, tai chi, and qigong bring such peace to the mind and body.

Let me tell you a short story about Rajat. Our Rajat bhaiya had hypertension, insulin resistance, and was forever stressed, working from 9 to 9, like most of us. Sab kuch tha except peace of mind. One fine day, he started attending yoga sessions just because his crush joined them (Typical desi jugaad, right?). Surprisingly, after a month, Rajat realized he wasn't just impressing his crush, but his blood pressure had dropped, and his sugar levels improved dramatically. Aur mood? Wah bhai wah, poora chill mode mein aa gaya! His anxiety levels had significantly reduced.

Science bolti hai, conditions like hypertension, insulin resistance, anxiety, depression, chronic pain, and cardiovascular issues can significantly improve with regular participation in mind-body exercises. According to research published in the Journal of Behavioral Medicine, activities such as tai chi and qigong have shown remarkable improvements in patients with chronic pain and stress-related conditions. Even hatha yoga's gentle poses contribute significantly towards managing anxiety and depression effectively.

Not only does it have peace of mind, but also these exercises genuinely enhance cognitive functions. You see, mind-body practices trigger neurological responses that strengthen your brain's neural pathways. Harvard Medical School studies confirm that regular meditation can literally alter your brain structure, enhancing memory, concentration, and overall cognitive abilities.

Now, what makes these exercises everyone's favourite? They are practical, portable, and low-intensity. Matlab, no need for heavy gym equipment or going to special studios, park mein jao, ghar pe karo, or even at your desk. Isse simple aur kya chahiye? This convenience and self-regulation make mind-body practices an ideal choice for busy individuals like you and me.

Aur ye hi nahi, these therapies also boost your balance, strength, and flexibility. Matlab sirf mental nahi, physical flexibility bhi full on, stretch karo aur khul ke jiyo! Whether it's your dadi practicing pranayama or your younger sibling doing surya namaskar before exams, the portability and simplicity appeal to every generation.

Here's a tip: Consistency is key. Regular, self-regulated mind-body practice is the real game-changer. So, folks, don't just read and nod; get up, stretch a bit, meditate a little, and unlock your own neurobiological magic!

In short, dost, mind-body connection ka funda simple hai, apna mind relax, toh body bhi mast! Incorporate these powerful practices into your daily life, and just like Rajat bhaiya, you'll soon be telling your own happy story.

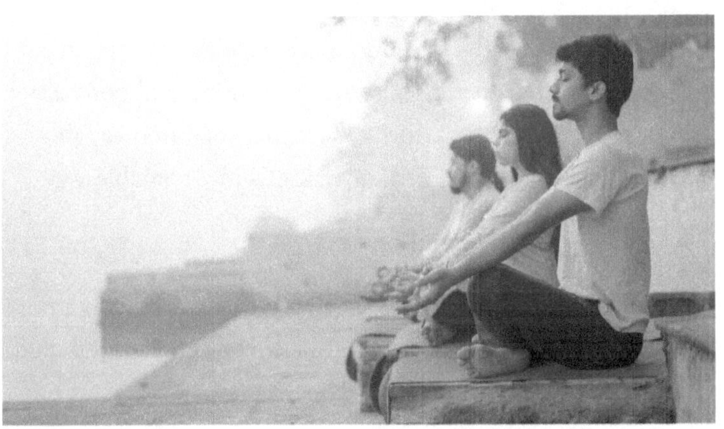

Quantum Healing, Awaken Your Inner Doctor

"Arre yaar, tum kitni dawa khaoge? Kabhi khud ko heal karne ka bhi try karo!" I laughed, half-serious, at my friend Ravi, who seemed eternally dependent on a cocktail of medicines. Ravi stared blankly, as if I'd just suggested he levitate.

"You think I'm some baba sitting in the Himalayas?" he retorted, rolling his eyes.

"Nahi bhai, but maybe Deepak Chopra can convince you!" I joked, passing him a copy of *Quantum Healing*. Little did I know, this casual exchange would alter the way I viewed my body, mind, and health forever.

Understanding Quantum Healing:

Quantum Healing, coined by the brilliant Dr. Deepak Chopra, emphasizes the body's innate ability to heal itself when aligned with the mind through meditation, visualization, and mindful practices. In simple terms, your mind and body aren't separate entities but partners in crime, together, capable of extraordinary feats. But let's unpack this in a relatable way.

The Body's Natural Intelligence:

Picture this: you accidentally slice your finger while chopping veggies. You don't sit around and manually instruct your skin, "Chalo bhaiya, jaldi se cells banalo!" Instead, your body automatically starts healing itself. This is your body's inbuilt wisdom, nature's autopilot mode.

Chopra describes how each cell in your body eavesdrops on your thoughts. Every time you think positively or negatively, your cells respond accordingly. It's like your body has a WhatsApp group where your mind constantly sends messages. Think good, empowering thoughts, and your body will reply with a thumbs-up. Think stressful thoughts, and your cells respond like those irritating forwarded messages that disrupt the group's harmony!

Mindfulness, Meditation, and Visualization:

Meditation isn't just for sadhus sitting cross-legged on mountains. It's a powerful tool anyone can use to tune into the body's innate healing mechanisms. Visualizing yourself healthy, imagining your body functioning optimally, actually helps your body to follow through. Chopra beautifully articulates that visualization is like giving your body a clear road map of where it needs to go. If you don't tell your cab driver your destination, how will he know where to take you?

I decided to test it myself. Once, during a particularly bad bout of fever, instead of endlessly popping pills, I took Chopra's advice. Closing my eyes, I visualized a warm golden light enveloping my body, flushing out toxins. Initially, I felt silly, but soon a strange calm overtook me. By evening, the fever had remarkably subsided without extra medication. Coincidence? Maybe. Quantum Healing? Definitely worth believing!

Scientific Backing and Research:

The skeptics among you (yes Ravi, talking to you!) will probably be thinking, this sounds like another dose of motivational gyaan. But here's where it gets real. Research from the Harvard Medical School and the American Psychological Association has confirmed that mindfulness and meditation significantly reduce stress and inflammation and improve overall well-being.

For instance, a study published in *JAMA Internal Medicine* showed mindfulness meditation could effectively reduce anxiety and depression, symptoms commonly associated with chronic illnesses. Another compelling research by neuroscientist Dr. Joe Dispenza demonstrated how regular visualization practices could influence physical health positively, such as improving immune response and speeding up recovery processes.

Deepak Chopra recounts numerous instances where patients, considered incurable by conventional medicine, experienced spontaneous remission through quantum healing techniques. Their stories aren't isolated. Even here in India, we've often heard stories of miraculous recoveries that baffle medical experts, this is Quantum Healing at play, tapping into the deep reservoirs of the mind-body connection.

Making Quantum Healing Your Own:

It's essential to integrate Quantum Healing into your life practically. Here are some steps to begin:

1. **Meditate Daily:** Even five minutes of mindfulness meditation can significantly impact your health.
2. **Positive Visualization:** Regularly visualize your body healing itself, especially if you're dealing with chronic issues.
3. **Watch Your Thoughts:** Remember, every thought is a message to your body. Keep those messages uplifting and positive.

"Ab toh convinced ho gaya?" I asked Ravi, after he tried Chopra's techniques and confessed feeling significantly better. He grinned sheepishly, "Haan, guruji, now I see my body as my friend, not an enemy."

Remember, your mind is more powerful than you think, your body smarter than you realize, and together, they are unstoppable. Let Quantum Healing be your secret superpower.

"SONA ZAROORI HAI BHAI!": THE SECRET WEAPON OF UNLIMITED ENERGY

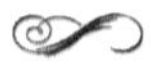

"If you don't make time for exercise, you'll probably have to make time for illness."

– Robin Sharma

If I had a rupee for every time someone told me, "Sleep is overrated, yaar. Life is for hustling," I'd probably have enough to sponsor everyone's melatonin supplements.

Let's face it, sleep has been underrated in our country for way too long. Late-night study sessions, binge-watching cricket highlights, endless Instagram reels, and yes, those midnight paratha cravings, we Indians have turned "sleep deprivation" into an unspoken badge of honor.

But let me tell you a hard truth: Sleep is not laziness. It is your body's *recharge button*, *detox centre*, *mood stabilizer*, and *focus enhancer*. It's the *desi jugaad* your body uses to keep you sane, sharp, and supercharged.

Without Sleep, Your Health Story Has No Happy Ending

Every organ, every emotion, every decision, depends on one basic habit: sleep. High-quality sleep doesn't just help you rest, it helps you *heal*. It restores organ function, balances hormones, boosts your brain, and powers up your energy system.

According to a global sleep survey, over **45% of people** are struggling to get enough sleep every night. And when sleep suffers, everything else begins to crumble, your work, your fitness, your mood, even your relationships.

Let me share a secret, everything that has ever helped me flourish started the night before, not the morning after.

Thousands of years ago, our ancestors lived in perfect harmony with nature. Sunrise meant it was time to hustle, hunting, gathering, making fires. And sunset? Time to wind down, cuddle into a cozy corner, and drift into deep, healing sleep.

Their internal clocks, called circadian rhythms, were guided by the rising and setting sun. Our DNA is still wired that way. But guess what happened?

Edison invented the bulb, and suddenly, light wasn't tied to the sun anymore. Then came TVs, laptops, mobile phones, and today, blue light is in our face even when it's midnight.

Now? We are working through the night, glued to screens, our pineal gland confused, and melatonin (our sleep hormone) suppressed like a junior intern in a board meeting.

Sleep Debt, it is the EMIs You're Paying Without Knowing

Here's what sleep deprivation does to your body:

- It **slows down your brain** (Judgment, perception, creativity, all gone).
- 17 hours of being awake = your brain behaves like it's had two glasses of wine.
- After 24 hours? Four glasses. Dangerous.
- It messes with your **weight, BP**, and **immune system**.
- It contributes to **mental health issues**, including **depression, anxiety**, and symptoms that mimic **ADHD**.

And it's not just about individual performance, major disasters like the **Challenger explosion, Chernobyl**, and the **Exxon Valdez oil spill** were linked to human error due to **lack of sleep**.

And in India? Ask any IT professional in Bengaluru burning the midnight oil for US calls, coffee keeps the body running, but the brain? Fried.

Are You Sleep Deprived? Be Honest!

Ask yourself:

- Do I wake up tired?
- Do I fall asleep during Netflix?
- Am I cranky without coffee?
- Do I feel low for no reason?

If yes, chances are you're not just tired, you're in **sleep debt**.

Let's take control. Let's bring structure to your sleep using *MacroHabits*, a set of repeatable rituals that sync your biological clock with the real world.

The Ideal Sleep Window:

Aim for **7.5 to 9 hours**. Research shows that between **10 PM and 6 AM** is when your body gets the richest REM (Rapid Eye Movement) sleep, when emotional healing and memory consolidation happen.

What happens when you skip this? You miss the brain's *clean-up duty*, and toxins that should have been flushed out stay back, clouding your focus the next day.

Let's break your 24-hour day into habits:

Morning:

- Wake up naturally, avoid alarms if possible.
- Get sunlight in your eyes within 30 minutes, triggers cortisol (the *good* stress hormone).
- No coffee post 12 PM. **Caffeine has a 6-hour half-life**. That's like eating pani puri at midnight and expecting no side effects.

Afternoon:

- If you're sleepy, take a **Power Nap (6–20 minutes)**. Anything more might make you groggy.
- Eat light, and move a little, take the stairs, stretch, breathe.

Evening:

- No exercise 4 hours before bedtime.
- Keep lights dim after sunset. Use warm yellow bulbs, not blinding white LEDs.
- Avoid social media scrollathons, they hijack your dopamine.

Twilight Hour (1 hour before bed):

- No emails, no WhatsApp.
- Journal, listen to calm music, or read.
- Use lavender oil or chamomile tea. Trust me, *dadi ke nuskhe* work wonders.
- Ensure complete darkness, use blackout curtains or eye masks.

The Sleep Sanctuary: Make Your Room a Temple of Rest

- Keep it cool (20°C or 68°F is ideal).
- Make it quiet: Use white noise if needed.
- Your bed = Only for sleep and love. No snacks, no Netflix marathons.
- Use calming colors: Soft pastels or earthy tones.
- Say no to clutter, clean room, clean mind.

When sleep isn't enough or isn't possible, use these:

Passive Rest (Naps):

- Power Nap (under 20 mins) for quick recovery.
- REM Nap (90+ mins) on weekends to deeply restore.

Active Rest:

- **Physical:** Stretch, deep breathing
- **Mental:** Meditation, gratitude journaling
- **Social:** Meaningful time with family/friends
- **Spiritual:** Prayer or mindfulness

These rituals calm your nervous system and help you sleep better at nig

Just like traffic rules, some sleep rules are sacred:

- No caffeine 8 hours before bed.
- No alcohol 3 hours before sleep, it wrecks REM.
- No large meals or desserts post 8 PM.
- No phones in bed, your sleep is not worth a meme.

Chris Bailey's *The Productivity Project* introduced this gem, **BPT** is when your brain is naturally most alert and focused. Find yours. Do your deepest work during BPT, and save the rest of the day for simpler tasks.

To find your BPT:

- Ditch sugar, caffeine, and alcohol for 3 weeks.
- Track your energy levels every hour.
- Use your peak hours for creative work.

That's how you work smarter, not longer, and make time for *The Golden Hour* of sleep.

Think of sleep as your *return on investment*. One extra hour of quality sleep can multiply your productivity, focus, and emotional resilience tenfold.

When you sleep better, you *live better*, and most importantly, you *love better*. Your work improves, your energy stays high, and you'll finally stop fighting with your partner over toothpaste caps.

Sleep is not an interruption in your day. It's the *engine that powers your life*. The quality of your sleep decides the quality of your thoughts, and your thoughts decide the quality of your actions, and ultimately, your life.

Don't wait till you crash to rest. Prioritize your *recovery like a CEO*, protect your sleep like a baby, and trust me, this one habit will help you rise like a phoenix.

Let's end with a promise: Tonight, we sleep not just to rest, but to rise. Tomorrow is going to be powerful.

So, set your alarm, not to wake up, but to *go to sleep*.

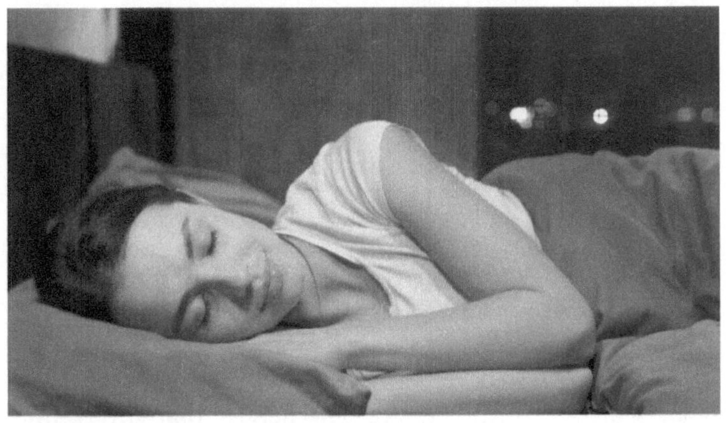

AYURVEDA: THE SECRET CODE OF VATA, PITTA, AND KAPHA

"When diet is wrong, medicine is of no use.
When diet is correct, medicine is of no need."

– Vasant Lad

This chapter is motivated by Vasant Lad's teachings in **Ayurveda: The Science of Self-Healing.**

Picture this, You wake up every morning either buzzing with ideas, feeling irritated by the heat, or refusing to leave your cozy blanket even at 10 AM.

Ever wondered **why your friend thrives on spicy biryani while your stomach screams murder?**

Or why you're super productive during winters while your buddy gets all sluggish?

Welcome to **Ayurveda's magic mirror,** the lens through which you finally understand YOUR BODY and what it wants.

Meet the Doshas: Vata, Pitta, and Kapha. These aren't just fancy Sanskrit words. They're bio-energies that govern how you look, feel, behave, digest food, react to stress, and even how you fall sick.

Each of us has a unique combination of all three, but one or two usually dominate.

Let's break it down like you're checking your own Jio plan.

VATA (Air + Ether)

The Creators. The Dreamers. The Fast Movers.

- Body: Thin frame, dry skin, cold hands and feet, quick walker
- Mind: Highly creative, quick to talk and think, but gets anxious easily
- Digestion: Irregular appetite, bloating, constipation
- Sleep: Light sleeper, often interrupted

PITTA (Fire + Water)

The Leaders. The Hotheads. The Focused Ones.

- Body: Medium build, warm body, reddish skin
- Mind: Intelligent, competitive, easily irritable
- Digestion: Strong appetite, heartburn or acidity
- Sleep: Moderate but light sleeper

KAPHA (Water + Earth)

The Lovers. The Loyal Ones. The Peacekeepers.

- Body: Sturdy frame, cool and oily skin, gains weight easily
- Mind: Calm, loving, but slow to get going
- Digestion: Slow digestion, loves sweets
- Sleep: Deep sleeper, snooze button expert

Eating wrong for your dosha is like using diesel in a petrol car. Disaster ahead.

VATA should avoid:

- Cold foods, raw salads, dry snacks like khakra
- Excessive caffeine, aerated drinks
- Too much movement, irregular meal timing

Best foods for Vata:

Warm, oily, grounding: like khichdi, ghee, milk, dates, warm soups.

PITTA should avoid:

- Spicy, fried, sour, salty foods: like achar, red chutney, rajma
- Alcohol, coffee, smoking
- Overworking or direct sun exposure

Best foods for Pitta:

Cooling, sweet, bitter: like cucumber, gulkand, mint, milk, coconut water.

KAPHA should avoid:

- Heavy, oily, sweet foods: like paneer, gulab jamun, wheat-based sweets
- Cold foods and drinks
- Oversleeping, lack of exercise

Best foods for Kapha:

Light, spicy, bitter: like moong dal, pepper rasam, green veggies, barley.

Balance is not about eating salad 3 times a day. It's about **syncing your routine with your inner engine.**

Vata Balancing Lifestyle

- Follow a fixed routine
- Warm oil massage with sesame oil
- Slow, grounding yoga
- Deep belly breathing and warm baths

Pitta Balancing Lifestyle

- Avoid peak heat (sun, heated arguments)
- Use coconut or sandalwood oil for massage
- Cooling pranayama (Sheetali)
- Sleep early, stay hydrated

Kapha Balancing Lifestyle

- Wake up before 6 AM
- Dry brushing and vigorous exercise
- Stimulating music, energizing yoga
- Avoid naps, eat light and early dinner

"Like increases Like. Opposites heal."

If you're a **fiery Pitta**, don't fuel it with more fire (spicy food, intense work). If you're a **cold, dry Vata**, avoid raw, cold salads. If you're a **slow Kapha**, move more and eat light.

You don't need to run to the Himalayas to balance your dosha. Just **understand who you are**, what your body wants, and give it that with love and regularity.

After all, the real journey is not just physical health: it's **Swabhav ke saath jeena.**

Live in tune with your nature.

What's Your Dosha?

Take the Quiz and Discover Your Ayurvedic Personality

Ⓐ VATA **Ⓑ PITTA** **Ⓒ KAPHA**

1. Body Frame & Weight

A) Thin, lanky, finds it hard to gain weight

B) Medium build, muscular, maintains weight easily

C) Broad, heavy build. gains weight easily

3. Hair

A) Dry, frizzy, thin

B) Straight, fine, may go grey early

C) Thick, oily, wavy

5. Digestion & Appetite

A) Irregular, may forget to eat

B) Strang hunger, gets irritable if meals are late

C) Slow digestion, feels heavy after eating

7. Reaction to Weather

A) Can't tolerate cold, prefers warmth

B) Can't tolerate heat, loves cool weather

C) Handles cold well, disiikes damp and cloudy days

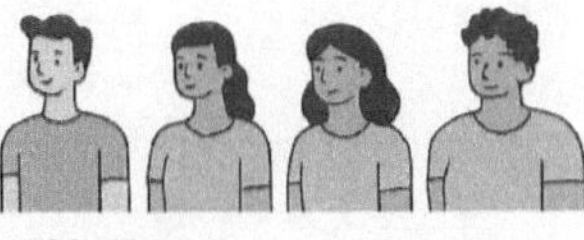

2. Skin Type

A) Dry, rough, tends to crack

B) Oily or reddish, sensitive to sun

C) Soft, pale, cool and moist

4. Sleep

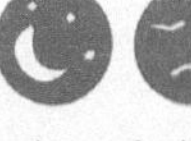 

A) Light, irregular, disturbed easily

B) Moderate, may wake up feeling hot

C) Deep, long, difficult to wake up

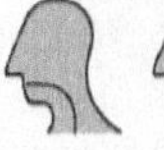 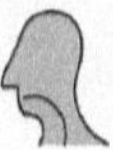 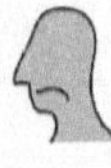 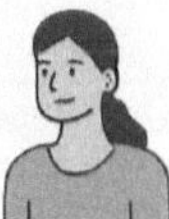

6. Personality & Mind

A) Creative, talkative, anxlous at times

B) Focused, driven, can get angry easily

C) Calm, loving, sometimes lazy or resistant to change

9. Energy Levels

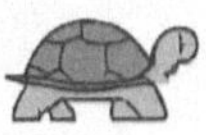

A) Variable — bursts of energy, then crashes

B) Strong and steady energy

C) Slow to start, but can go on for long

Scoring System:

Count how many times you chose:

- **A = VATA**
- **B = PITTA**
- **C = KAPHA**

Your Result:

Mostly A: You are VATA dominant!

Mostly B: You are PITTA dominant!

Mostly C: You are KAPHA dominant!

STAY

FABULOUS

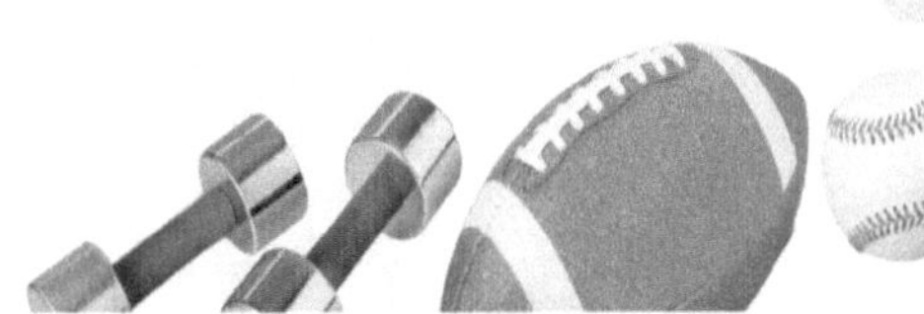

SABSE BADA ROG, KYA KAHENGE LOG!!

"Your health account, your bank account, they're the same thing. The more you put in, the more you can take out."

- Jack LaLanne

Let me tell you a quick story. Back in college, I once walked into the campus wearing bright blue chinos. I thought I looked dope. Like, Ranveer Singh-level swag. But the moment I stepped into the canteen, I felt like everyone turned to look at me. My brain screamed, "Bro, sab dekh rahe hain!" And I immediately regretted my fashion choice.

That whole day, I avoided people, skipped a lecture, and even ate lunch alone behind the library. For what? Because I *thought* people were judging me. Truth is? No one cared. Everyone was busy being the hero of their own drama. That's when I learned about the *spotlight effect*, we think everyone's watching us, but they're not. They're too busy worrying about how they look.

Cut to today: I still wear those blue chinos. And this time, I own them.

Let's Talk Bukowski: The OG "I Dont Give A F*ck" Guy

Mark Manson starts his book with Charles Bukowski, a drunk, broke, messed-up dude who, despite being rejected all his life, went on to become a best-selling author. Why? Because he never pretended. He accepted he was a loser and wrote honestly about it. His tombstone says: "Don't try." And that's the essence, stop pretending to be someone you're not just to please people.

In a world where everyone's chasing validation, more likes, more swipes, more approvals, the biggest rebellion is to say, "I'm cool with who I am."

Confidence Is Not in the Mirror, It's in the Mind

If you have to stand in front of a mirror and say "I am confident" 10 times, bhai, you're not. Just like happy people don't go around shouting "I'm happy!", real confidence doesn't make noise.

It's like Manson says: the desire for more positive experiences is itself a negative experience. You keep saying, "I want to be confident," because deep down, you believe you're not. Flip it. Say, "I may not be perfect, but I still choose to show up."

Give a F*ck, But Choose Wisely

In India, people will give you advice even if you don't ask. Sharma uncle will tell you you're too thin, Renu aunty will ask when you're getting married, and your old school friend will DM you, "Bro, you've changed."

Here's the secret: it's not about giving zero f*cks. *It's about giving f*cks to things that matter.* Your health? Yes. Your purpose? Yes. Sharma uncle's opinion? Hard pass.

Manson puts it beautifully: "You only have a limited number of f*cks to give. *So you must choose your f*cks wisely.*"

The Feedback Loop from Hell

Ever felt anxious about feeling anxious? Or felt bad because you're feeling low? That's the *feedback loop from hell.* And trust me, a lot of us live there rent-free.

I used to overthink every mistake. "What will people think?" "What if I fail?" "Will they laugh?" One day, after messing up a work presentation, I just said: "Haan bhai, galti hui. So what?" That night, I slept like a baby.

Accept that you'll mess up. That's life. That's growth. That's how you build real confidence, not by avoiding failure, but by facing it without shame.

Bro Tip: Be Comfortable Being Different

Confidence isn't loud. It's silent. It's sitting in a room full of people, all trying to fit in, and you sitting there, chilling in your truth. Maybe you're the guy who doesn't drink at parties. Maybe you prefer building your side hustle on weekends instead of clubbing. Maybe you love wearing kurtas in a world chasing sneakers. Good! Own it.

Because the moment you stop needing others to validate your choices, you become free.

The Indian Twist: Inner Peace Over Outer Show

We Indians are culturally conditioned to seek approval. "Log kya kahenge" is a whole vibe. But guess what? "Log" are just as confused as you. So instead of dancing to everyone else's tune, ask yourself: *What matters to me?*

Want to dance in the rain? Do it. Want to start over at 30? Start. Want to wear a dhoti with sneakers? Style it, bhai!

Confidence doesn't come from being the loudest in the room. It comes from being unapologetically you, quiet, consistent, and clear.

So, next time you walk into a room wondering if people are judging you, remember: they're too busy judging themselves. Smile. Sit straight. Speak your truth.

And if all else fails, wear those blue chinos again.

Because confidence isn't about them. It's about you. And when you finally stop giving f*cks about being liked, you start living a life you actually like.

HOW TO WEAR YOUR STYLEEEE!!

"If it doesn't challenge you, it won't change you."

– Fred DeVito

I know this struggle firsthand. When you're carrying extra weight, **dressing up feels like a battle.**

Every outfit feels wrong. **Jeans are tight on the thighs, T-shirts stick to the belly, and formal shirts never sit right on the shoulders.** It feels like clothes were made for a different species altogether.

And the worst part? The constant self-consciousness.

The Joke That Changed Everything

I still remember **one incident in Kota** during my IIT prep days. I was walking past a group of girls, minding my own business, when one of them joked to her friend, **"Arre dekh, tera boyfriend ja raha hai!"**

It was meant to be funny, but *bhai*, that cut deep. I wasn't just overweight; I felt invisible, and when people did notice me, it was for all the wrong reasons.

That day, something clicked. Instead of **hiding behind oversized, loose-fitting clothes,** I started observing **what fashionable people did differently.** And **slowly, I cracked the code of dressing well, even with extra weight.**

So, if you're stuck thinking **"Nothing looks good on me"**, let me help you **fix that mindset and your wardrobe.** Because **no matter your size, you can look sharp, stylish, and damn confident.**

STYLING FOR WOMEN:

DRESS FOR YOUR BODY TYPE

Women's fashion is full of trends, but the real **secret to looking good isn't wearing what's trendy, it's wearing what suits your body.**

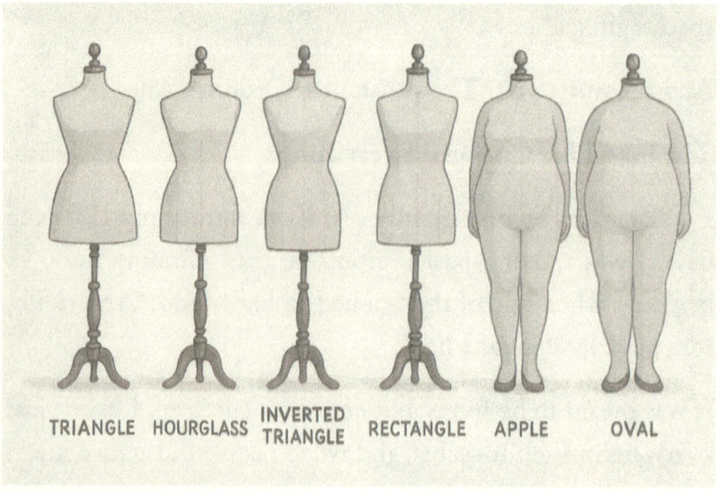

1) TRIANGLE BODY TYPE (Pear-Shaped)

(*Hips wider than shoulders, weight centered around hips*)

Your Goal: Balance your silhouette by drawing attention upwards.

Celeb Example: Deepika Padukone (*before she got ripped for Pathaan*).

What Works:

- Jackets that end **above or below the hips** to avoid emphasizing them.
- Structured **shoulder details** (puffed sleeves, wide necklines).
- Dark, plain-colored pants to slim down the lower body.

Avoid:

- Skirts or pants with big pockets (makes the hips look even wider).
- Heavy embroidery around the hip area.

2) HOURGLASS BODY TYPE

(*Shoulders and hips balanced, well-defined waist*)

Your Goal: Highlight your natural proportions **without ruining the balance.**

Celeb Example: Priyanka Chopra, Aishwarya Rai (*classic hourglass queens*).

What Works:

- **Wrap dresses, belted outfits, high-waisted trousers** to show off your waist.
- **V-neck, square neck tops** to enhance the natural shape.

Avoid:

- **Turtlenecks and boxy outfits** (they kill the curves).
- **Baggy or oversized clothes** (they hide your best asset, your waist!).

3) INVERTED TRIANGLE BODY TYPE

(Broad shoulders, narrower hips, athletic build)

Your Goal: Soften the top half and create volume below.

Celeb Example: Anushka Sharma (*she naturally has broad shoulders*).

What Works:

- A-line skirts, **flowy palazzo pants** to add volume to the lower body.
- **Deep V-neck tops** (they balance wide shoulders).
- **Belts** to define the waist and create curves.

Avoid:

- Shoulder pads (*unless you want to look like a football player*).
- High-neck tops that make the shoulders look broader.

4) APPLE BODY TYPE

(*Weight in the upper body, rounder belly, slim legs*)

Your Goal: Draw attention away from the tummy and towards your legs.

Celeb Example: Vidya Balan (*she embraces flowy outfits that work for her*).

What Works:

- **V-neck tops** (elongate your torso and make you look slimmer).
- **A-line dresses, structured jackets, flowy tunics.**
- **Straight-cut pants** that show off slim legs.

Avoid:

- **Belts or tight-fitting tops** (they emphasize the midsection).
- **Heavy patterns around the belly area.**

5) OVAL BODY TYPE

(*Weight is evenly spread, undefined waist*)

Your Goal: Create structure and shape.

Celeb Example: Oprah Winfrey (*she nails structured outfits!*).

What Works:

- **Long, structured blazers and vertical stripes.**
- **Dark-colored outfits with pops of color in accessories.**

Avoid:

- **Baggy outfits that add unnecessary bulk.**
- **Bright patterns around the midsection.**

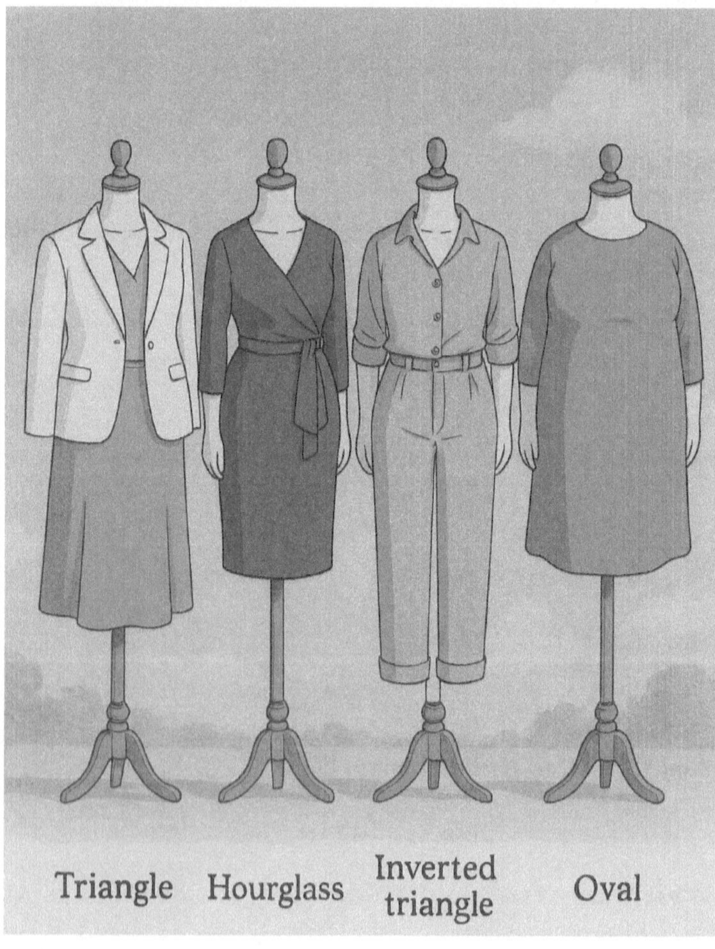

STYLING FOR MEN: LOOK POWERFUL, NOT SLOPPY

Men's fashion is simpler than women's, but that doesn't mean **you can throw on anything and call it a day.**

Rule #1: A Well-Tailored Suit Is to Women What Lingerie Is to Men

Ever seen **Ranveer Singh in a tuxedo?** Forget the quirky outfits, when he wears a classic **black tux**, it screams **power, money, and confidence.**

Why? Because **fit matters more than size.**

If you're overweight, **STOP buying oversized clothes thinking they'll hide the fat.** Instead, buy **well-fitted** clothes that structure your body.

MEN'S BODY TYPES & HOW TO DRESS

1) THE TRIANGLE BODY (Most Overweight Men)

(*Wider waist, narrower shoulders*)

Your Goal: Create a V-shape illusion.

Celeb Example: Boman Irani (*He wears structured jackets to balance his shape*).

What Works:

- **Dark, structured blazers** to broaden the shoulders.
- **V-neck shirts** to elongate the torso.

Avoid:

- Tightly fitted shirts (*they highlight belly fat*).
- Round-neck T-shirts (*makes the upper body look even bulkier*).

2) RECTANGLE BODY (Straight Frame, No Definition)

Your Goal: Add shape.

Celeb Example: Shahid Kapoor.

What Works:

- **Layering** (blazers, open shirts over T-shirts).
- **Slim-fit shirts** to create a structured frame.

Avoid:

- Oversized T-shirts (*they make you look boxy*).
- Flat-front pants (*adds no shape*).

3) INVERTED TRIANGLE BODY (Athletic Build, Broad Shoulders)

Your Goal: Balance your proportions.

Celeb Example: Hrithik Roshan (*his stylist knows how to play up his shoulders*).

What Works:

- **V-neck T-shirts** that don't add bulk to the shoulders.
- **Straight-leg pants** (keeps things proportional).

Avoid:

- Shoulder-padded blazers (*you don't need more bulk*).
- Ultra-tight T-shirts (*makes the chest look too top-heavy*).

MEN'S STYLE COMMANDMENTS

- ✔ **Get the right fit.** Tailor your clothes if needed.
- ✔ **Ditch baggy clothes.** They make you look bigger.
- ✔ **Invest in quality fabrics.** A cheap shirt looks cheap.
- ✔ **Dark colors slim you down.** A well-fitted black outfit = instant 10kg fat loss.
- ✔ **Shoes matter.** Sneakers for casual, loafers for smart casual, and Oxfords for formal.

STYLE IS NOT ABOUT SIZE

At the end of the day, **style is an observational skill.** You **don't** need to lose 20kg to look good. You just need the **right fit, right fabrics, and right confidence.**

So go out there, **own your look,** and let the world see **the stylish YOU,** no matter what the scale says.

Confidence is Your Best Outfit

Do you ever walk into a room and spot that one guy who **just looks like he owns the place**? He's got the right posture, a well-fitted blazer, and a crisp shirt that screams, *I make money while you blink.*

Now, here's the thing, **he may or may not actually be successful.** But because he **looks** the part, people **assume** he is. That's the **Halo Effect**, when you dress well, people **automatically assign you higher status, wealth, and intelligence.**

And the best part? **You don't need six-pack abs or a model face to pull this off.** You just need the right outfit and **the confidence to own it.**

Why Style = Power (Even When You're Overweight)

Most overweight guys believe that **style isn't for them.** They think, *"I'll start dressing well after I lose weight."*

That's where they go wrong.

When you dress sharp, **you feel sharp**. And when you feel sharp, **you act sharp.** You walk differently. You talk differently. People notice you differently.

Even **businessmen and CEOs** understand this. Think about it, why do successful men wear suits? Not just because it looks good, but because it **commands respect.**

Ever seen Mukesh Ambani in a sloppy outfit? **Never.** Because he knows **dressing well is a power move.**

Even if you're overweight, the right outfit can **redefine your presence** in a room. **So stop hiding behind baggy T-shirts and track pants.** Step up your game, and people will treat you accordingly.

3 Key Looks for Every Guy

Not every occasion demands a suit, and not every day is casual. You need a **versatile wardrobe** that works across different situations while keeping you stylish.

Here's a simple breakdown of **three essential looks** that every man (especially if you're carrying extra weight) should master.

1. Classic (Formal & Business): Power Dressing

Best For: Office, weddings, business meetings, high-end restaurants

The Key: A well-tailored suit is the biggest game-changer for overweight men. Forget fast fashion, **get your suit tailored.**

Color Palette: Stick to **black, navy, charcoal grey.**

Fit Matters: No loose sleeves, no saggy pants. **Go slim, not tight.**

Shirts: Classic **white, light blue, or pastel shades** (avoid shiny fabrics).

Shoes: Black or brown leather Oxfords (never cheap synthetic ones).

Accessories: A clean, minimal watch (leave the bling to rappers).

Why It Works?

- **A dark suit slims you down instantly.**
- A **structured blazer** balances your proportions.
- **People automatically take you more seriously.**

✔ **Celeb Inspiration:**

- **Virat Kohli** (*when he steps into a boardroom, he's always power-dressed*).
- **Shah Rukh Khan** (*classic black suits, always sophisticated*).

2. Smart Casual: Effortless Elegance

Best For: Dinner dates, office outings, social events, semi-formal occasions

The Key: Smart casual is about looking **put-together, without going full corporate mode.** It's **relaxed yet stylish.**

Blazer: Navy blue, beige, or grey

Shirt: Well-fitted button-down in **white, light blue, or soft prints**

Pants: Chinos or tailored trousers (ditch the jeans here)

Shoes: Loafers or brogues (brown or black)

Accessories: A leather belt that matches your shoes

Why It Works?

- The **blazer shapes your body**, making you look more structured.
- Chinos **are comfortable yet polished.**
- Perfect for **networking, dating, and work events** without looking overdressed.

✔ **Celeb Inspiration:**

- **Ranbir Kapoor** (*perfectly nails the blazer + chino look*).
- **Hrithik Roshan** (*even in casual mode, always put-together*).

3. Casual: Everyday Style, Without Looking Basic

Best For: Brunch, movie nights, casual meetups, travel

The Key: Casual doesn't mean sloppy.

Jeans: Dark blue, straight fit (NEVER baggy, NEVER skinny)

T-shirt/Polo: Solid colors work best, **black, white, navy, olive, maroon**

Sneakers: White leather sneakers or clean trainers

Jackets: Denim or lightweight bomber jackets

Accessories: A good watch, sunglasses, and a minimal bracelet (optional)

Why It Works?

- **Dark jeans + fitted T-shirt = instant slimming effect.**
- **A polo shirt is a great upgrade from regular T-shirts.**
- Sneakers keep it casual but **clean and modern.**

✔ **Celeb Inspiration:**

- **Vicky Kaushal** (*classic casual done right*).
- **Farhan Akhtar** (*effortless cool with basic yet stylish outfits*).

Own Your Look, Own Your Presence

Here's the ultimate truth: **The world sees you the way you present yourself.**

You don't need **expensive brands**. You don't need **a model's body. You just need the right fit, right fabrics, and the confidence to own your style.**

The next time you step out, don't just wear clothes. **Wear your presence.** Because **confidence is your best outfit, and it never goes out of style.**

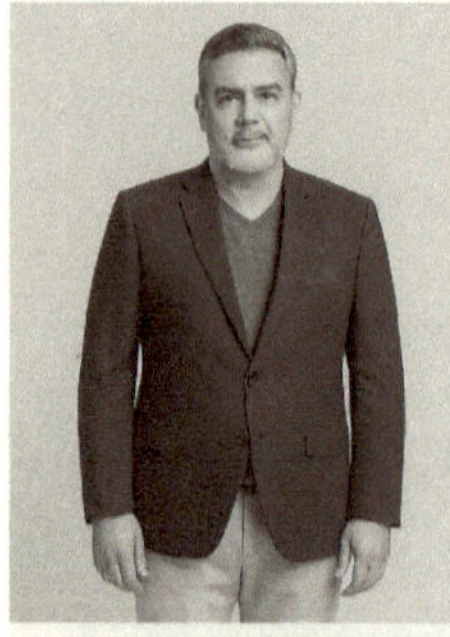

THE TRIANGLE BODY
(Most Overweight Men)
Your Goal: Create V-shape illuston.
Celeb Example: Boman Irani (He wears structured jackets to balance his shape)
What Works: Dark, structurred blazers to broaden the shoulders.

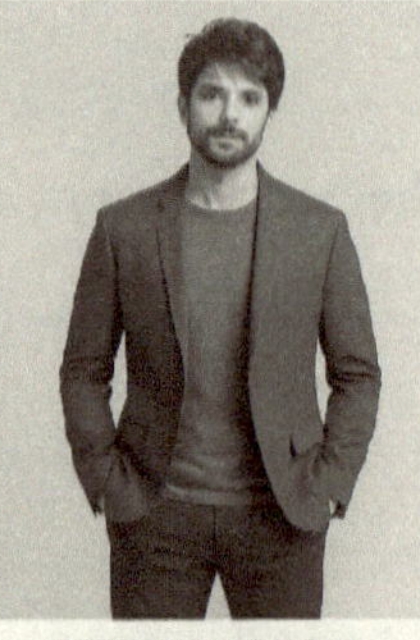

RECTANGLVE BODY
(Ctraight Frame)
Your Goal: Add shape.
Celeb Example: Shahid
What Works: Layering (blazers, open shirts over T-Shirts)
Avoid: Oversized T-shirts (they make li ke u ldck boxy,

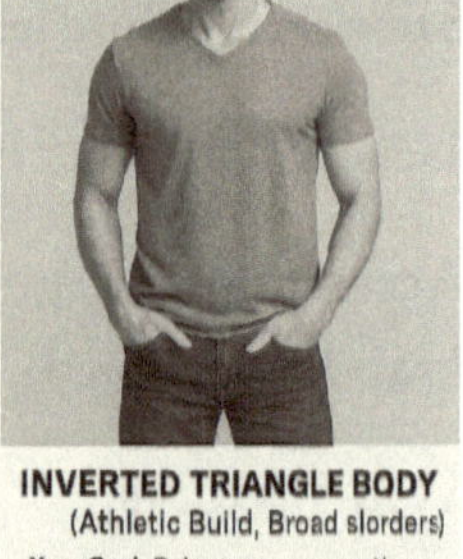

INVERTED TRIANGLE BODY
(Athletic Build, Broad slorders)
Your Goal: Balance yur proportions.
Celeb Example: Hrithik Roshan (his stylist knows how to play up sis
Avoid: Schoulder-padded blazers
Ultra-tight T-Shirts: (makes the dnest) look tas top-heavy)

WHERE DID MY MUSCLES GO? THE AGING MUSCLE MYSTERY

There was a time in my 20s when lifting a gas cylinder at home was my casual warm-up. Now, after I crossed 30, even changing the water can feels like deadlifting a bike. Sound familiar?

As we grow older, something strange happens, not overnight, but slowly, silently, and sneakily. Our muscles start saying, *"Bhai, bas ho gaya, ab rest chahiye."* And this is where the story of aging muscles, or what fancy scientists call **Sarcopenia** (Greek for "loss of flesh"), begins.

If Only We Were Bears…

Imagine this: it's freezing cold, and like a boss, you hibernate like a bear, no work, no gym, no cardio. You sleep for months and wake up fresh, without losing any muscle.

But alas, we are not bears.

Humans, unlike our furry mountain friends, **lose muscle mass shockingly fast** when we become inactive. Even just **three weeks of bed rest** can shrink your leg muscles by **10%**. Now think about astronauts, floating in space without gravity, they lose **20% of their muscle mass** in **just one to two weeks**.

And here's the catch, *aging does the same thing*, just at a slower pace. The tragedy? It's often ignored.

The Great Muscle Heist of Old Age

Growing old is not just about greying hair or forgetting where you kept your phone. One of the biggest threats of aging is **losing muscle strength and function**, a condition so silent yet so dangerous, it deserves a warning sign.

Let's talk real stats:

- In the US and UK, **grip strength** (a great indicator of overall muscle health) **declines by 25%** between age 25 and 75.
- A study from **Framingham, Massachusetts** found that among women aged 75-84, **65% couldn't lift 10 pounds** (around 4.5 kg), that's like lifting a baby!
- Climbing stairs, getting off a chair, or even walking normally becomes a mission impossible.

And the worst part? The weaker you get, the **less you move**, and the less you move, the **weaker you become**, a vicious cycle that can ruin your golden years.

Sarcopenia: The Silent Epidemic in Every Indian Household

If you're thinking *"Yeh sab foreign logon ke studies hain, India mein toh sab theek hai"*, then let's pause.

In India, with increasing urbanization, sedentary jobs, and reliance on domestic help, our seniors are **equally or more vulnerable**. The National Programme for Health Care of the Elderly (Govt. of India) has noted increasing physical disabilities due to **muscle loss, lack of exercise, and poor nutrition** among our aging population.

While our *nana-nani* or *dada-dadi* may not call it "sarcopenia," they often say, *"Ab taaqat nahi rahi beta."*

Far away in the Amazon, the **Aché tribe** lives like our ancient ancestors, walking, hunting, cooking on their own, every single day. You know what's surprising? A 70-year-old Aché woman has the **same grip strength** as a 50-year-old woman in England!

That's the secret of staying active.

And no, it's not about running marathons. It's about **moving your body with purpose**, lifting your own things, walking to the market, and keeping your muscles alive.

Muscles Are Not Dead, They're Just Sleeping: Wake Them Up! Here's the best part of the story, **you can reverse this process**. Yes, even if you are 80!

Multiple studies, including one published in *JAMA (Journal of the American Medical Association)*, show that **resistance training** (basic weight lifting) can **increase muscle size and strength** in people aged 87–96.

And it doesn't mean you need to join a hardcore gym.

- Lifting water bottles.
- Doing chair squats.
- Resistance bands at home.

- Climbing stairs instead of using lifts.

Simple things, done daily, can help muscles **bounce back** like college kids after an energy drink.

Muscles Save More Than Just Pride: They Save Your Life

When your muscles go, they take your health with them.

- **Osteoporosis** (weak bones)? Your muscles weren't loading the bones enough.
- **Heart disease** and **Type 2 Diabetes**? Your body wasn't burning enough sugar due to inactivity.
- **Falls and injuries?** Weak muscles can't support you during imbalance.

And perhaps the most underrated impact, **depression**. Exercise, especially strength training, **releases feel-good hormones**, boosts self-esteem, and reduces symptoms of anxiety and depression. A 2020 meta-analysis from Harvard confirmed this, **strength training is like therapy for the mind**.

India Needs a Muscle Revolution for Its Elders

Our elderly don't need just medicines. They need **muscle therapy**.

Imagine:

- Senior parks with resistance machines.
- Evening community sessions for strength training.
- Diet plans to include more **protein** for muscle recovery.

- Families encouraging their elders to *walk, stretch, and lift,* instead of saying, *"Arre beta, mat karo. Thak jaoge."*

Muscles are **not just for bodybuilders or young influencers.** They're for **every human being who wants to live with dignity and strength.**

The Final Thought: Your Muscles Remember You

Muscles have memory. They don't forget how strong you once were. All they ask is, *"Yaad rakhoge toh wapas aa jaayenge."*

So whether you're 35 or 85, it's never too late to pick up that dumbbell, carry that grocery bag, or walk that extra kilometre.

Let your body know that you haven't given up. Because *"zindagi lambi ho ya chhoti, taqat ke saath jeeyo."*

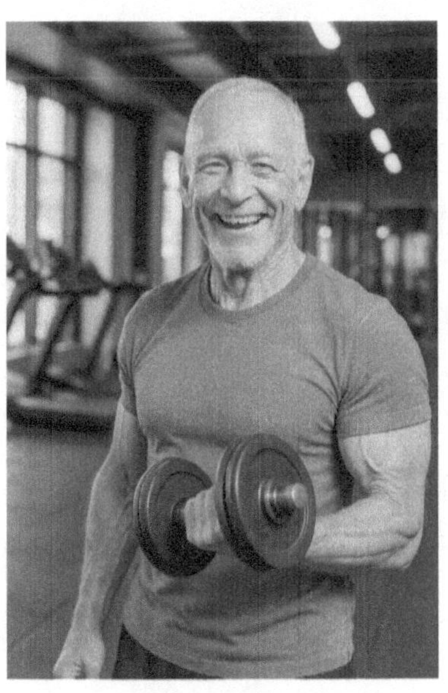

"Kuch karna hai, par motivation nahi aa raha."

If you've ever said this to yourself while staring at a blank wall, waiting for some magical force to push you into action, welcome to the club.

Building healthy habits isn't about waking up one fine morning with an unstoppable drive to hit the gym or eat clean. It's about tricking your mind into doing something so consistently that it becomes second nature. And what better way to do that than by turning it into a challenge?

Challenges make things exciting. They give us structure, a goal, and, most importantly, the sweet dopamine hit of achievement. Here are some of the most popular types of challenges that can help you build the habit of health. Pick your fighter!

1. The 21-Day Challenge (Because We All Love a Good Shortcut)

You've heard the golden rule, "It takes 21 days to form a habit." While the science behind it is debatable, there's no denying that committing to something for three weeks is a solid way to get started.

The idea is simple: choose one small, achievable habit (like drinking 3 liters of water daily, doing 10 push-ups, or avoiding junk food) and stick to it for 21 days.

What happens next? Two things, either your body adapts, and it becomes effortless, or you at least get past the hardest part: the beginning.

For example, I had a friend who was struggling to wake up early. He started a **21-day '5 AM Club' challenge.** The first week? Torture. The second week? Less painful. By the third week, waking up early felt normal. It didn't mean he never slept in again, but he now had a default habit he could rely on.

2. The 75 Hard Challenge (The Boss Level Mode)

If you think 21 days is for rookies, meet **75 Hard.** This challenge is NOT for the faint-hearted. It involves:

- Two workouts a day (one must be outdoors, no excuses)
- Drinking a gallon of water daily
- Reading 10 pages of a self-improvement book
- Following a strict diet (no cheat meals, no alcohol)
- Taking a daily progress photo

The catch? **Miss even one rule, and you start from Day 1.**

Sounds extreme? It is. But it also builds insane mental toughness. I've seen people who started this just to get fit but ended up feeling like different human beings by the end of it, more disciplined, more confident, and with a 'no excuses' mindset.

Think of it as your **military boot camp, but without an angry sergeant screaming at you.**

3. The 10,000 Steps Challenge (The OG Movement Hack)

This one's for those who feel like exercise is *too much effort*. Just walk, **10,000 steps a day, every day.**

Walking is underrated. It improves cardiovascular health, burns calories, reduces stress, and helps digestion. Plus, it doesn't require a gym membership or expensive shoes (though investing in a comfy pair won't hurt).

The best part? You can make it fun, listen to podcasts, talk to a friend, or just take a break from screen time. Some people have even turned this into a **'Evening Chai Walk' challenge**, where they only allow themselves a cup of tea if they've completed 10,000 steps.

A little desi twist never hurts!

4. The No Sugar Challenge (Sweetness with a Side of Pain)

Sugar is the villain we all love. It's everywhere, chai, biscuits, namkeen, that 'one bite' of cake at office birthdays. And once it's in your system, your body keeps craving more.

A **No Sugar Challenge** helps break that cycle. It means cutting out all forms of processed sugar, no desserts, no sugary drinks, no hidden sugars in packaged foods, for a set number of days (usually 30).

Most people who try this experience crazy withdrawal symptoms initially, headaches, mood swings, and an unexplainable urge to murder anyone eating chocolate in front of them. But if you survive the first few weeks, you'll notice:

- More energy
- Better skin
- Less bloating
- Fewer random cravings

And when you finally eat something sweet again, it actually tastes *too* sweet. That's when you realize how much your body has adapted.

5. The Cold Shower Challenge (Because Comfort is Overrated)

Now, this one is more about **mental toughness** than physical health. Taking a **cold shower every day for 30 days** sounds like some medieval torture, but it has surprising benefits, improving blood circulation, boosting immunity, and increasing alertness.

More importantly, it trains your brain to **embrace discomfort**.

The first few times, your body will scream, **"Bhai, why?!"** But soon, you'll realize something powerful, you're in control. You can do things that seem difficult. And once you apply this mindset to other areas of life, you start seeing change.

6. The Intermittent Fasting Challenge (Modern Fasting, Without the Religion)

This is one of the most effective challenges for **weight loss and metabolic health**. The idea is simple: eat within a fixed window (e.g., 8 hours) and fast for the remaining time.

Popular versions include:

- **16:8 fasting** (16 hours fast, 8 hours eating window)
- **OMAD (One Meal A Day)**
- **5:2 fasting (5 normal days, 2 low-calorie days)**

IF isn't just about **when** you eat but also about **how it resets your body.** It helps regulate insulin, improves digestion, and even boosts brain function.

Just one tip, **don't use it as an excuse to binge on biryani and pastries in your eating window.**

7. The No Screens Before Bed Challenge (Save Your Sleep, Save Your Brain)

Scrolling on your phone till 2 AM and then wondering why you wake up like a zombie? Welcome to the age of **dopamine overdose.**

This challenge is about **no screens at least 1 hour before bedtime.** No Instagram, no WhatsApp debates, no YouTube rabbit holes. Instead, replace it with:

- Reading a book
- Journaling

- Meditating
- Just lying in bed (yes, doing nothing is a skill)

It might feel unnatural at first (because, let's be honest, scrolling is our generation's lullaby), but after a week, you'll notice deeper sleep and better mornings.

WHICH CHALLENGE WILL YOU TAKE?

At the end of the day, **challenges are just a way to trick your brain into consistency.** The real game is about showing up daily, even when you don't feel like it.

So, what's stopping you? Pick a challenge, commit to it, and see how your body (and mind) transforms.

And remember, **the hardest part is starting. Once you begin, you're already winning.**

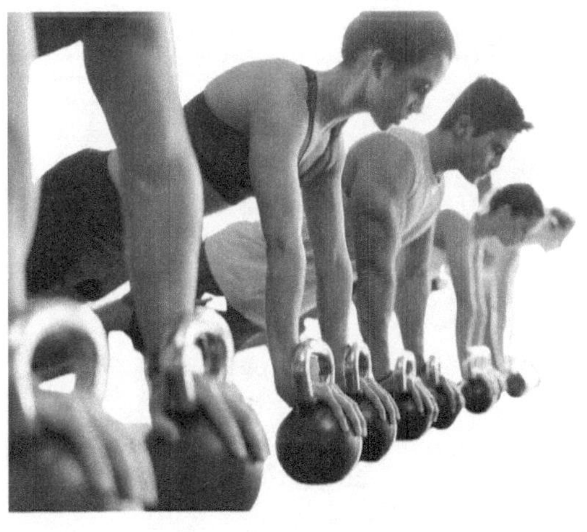

HOW DO I READ THE LABELS ON PRODUCTS?

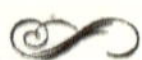

"A fit body, a calm mind, a house full of love, these things cannot be bought, they must be earned."

– Naval Ravikant

Nutrition Facts

Serving Size: 30g (About 1 small bowl)

Serving Per Serving

Calories   **145**

Calories 145 kcal		7%
Saturated Fat		5%
Trans Fat		0%
Unsaturated Fat		4%
Cholesterol 0 mg		0%
Sodium 180 mg		8%
Total Carbohydrate 18 g		6%
Dietary Fiber 4 g		16%
Total Sugars 2 g		2%
Added Sugars 1 g		2%
Protein 7 g		14%

Calcium 50 mg	4%	Iron	1,2 mg	10%
Vitamin B12	10%	Vitamin B12		20%

Ingredients: Multigrian flour (millet, oats, wheat), chickpea protein, sunflower oil, pink salt, dehydratedjg garlic, onion powder, black pepper, turmeric, natural flavors, no preservatives, no artifical colors

According to an **FSSAI survey** (India), 62% of urban consumers do **not** read labels fully. A study in *The Journal of Consumer Affairs* (2021) found people who regularly read labels had **lower BMI** and better **nutritional awareness**. WHO suggests front-of-package labeling could reduce obesity if people make informed decisions.

Reading labels isn't about paranoia. It's about **self-respect**.

You work hard, earn money, and make time to eat. So why not eat something that gives you energy, not diseases?

We all know the drill.

You're in a supermarket, clutching a shiny packet of *multigrain chips* or *low-fat yogurt*. The front label screams things like **"high protein," "organic," "zero sugar"**, and you're thinking, *"Bas, this is healthy!"*

But here's the deal. The real story? It's written on the back. In fine print. In science-y words. That most of us either ignore or don't understand.

But not anymore.

This chapter is your torchlight into the world of food labels. Because when you know **what to look for**, you'll never be fooled by fancy packaging again. Let's decode this like a pro. Not for the sake of looking smart, but to **actually become smarter about your health.**

1. Start With the Serving Size: The Sneakiest Trick in the Book

First line. First trap.

"Serving Size: 28g (1/2 cup), Servings Per Container: 4"

You see 120 calories and think, *"Not bad."* But wait, are you eating **just 1 serving** or the **whole pack**?

Most of us eat the whole thing and unknowingly double, triple, or even quadruple the calories. **Always multiply by the number of servings you'll actually eat.** This one hack will change your entire perspective.

2. Calories: The Energy Currency

Calories aren't evil. They're just energy.

But here's where things get real: what **kind** of calories are you getting?

- 200 calories from **walnuts** ≠ 200 calories from **potato chips**
- One gives **nutrients**, the other gives **inflammation**

Focus less on just *how many* calories and more on *where they're coming from.*

3. Sugar: The Sweet Poison

Sugar hides in more costumes than a Bollywood villain. It's not just listed as "sugar."

Look for:

- **Dextrose**
- **High fructose corn syrup**
- **Maltose**
- **Fruit concentrate**
- **Caramel syrup**

Pro tip: If sugar is in the **first 3 ingredients**, run! It means it's a **major ingredient**.

Also, check for **Added Sugars** under Total Sugars. That's the culprit for fat gain, hormonal imbalances, and that mid-afternoon slump you feel post-lunch.

4. Sodium: A Silent Sinner

India is already high in BP cases. And guess what? Most of the sodium doesn't come from your salt shaker, it comes from processed food.

A healthy adult should consume **less than 2,300 mg** sodium daily (about 1 tsp of salt)

But just one packet of instant noodles can have up to **1,200 mg!**

High sodium = water retention + bloating + hypertension = Dard hi Dard

5. Ingredients List: Your Truth Teller

This is the most **underrated** but **most powerful** part of the label.

Follow this golden rule:

"Shorter the list, the better the product."

If you see 25 ingredients, and you can't pronounce half of them, chances are, your body won't recognize them either.

Avoid:

- **Artificial colors**
- **Preservatives like BHA, BHT**
- **MSG (monosodium glutamate)**
- **Hydrogenated oils** (a.k.a. trans fat)

First 3 ingredients = What the product mostly contains

If it starts with *wheat flour, sugar, palm oil*, that "protein bar" is basically a dessert.

6. Fats: Don't Fear, Just Know Them

Fats have a bad reputation. But not all fats are bad.

Understand the three:

- **Good Fats:** Unsaturated fats (found in nuts, seeds, olive oil)
- **Moderate Fats:** Saturated fats (found in butter, ghee, meat)
- **Bad Fats:** Trans fats (found in fried junk, baked goods with "hydrogenated" oils)

If a label says **0g trans fat** but has *partially hydrogenated oil* in ingredients, **they're lying**. Legally, if it's less than 0.5g, they can say 0. But even that much daily can hurt your heart.

7. Protein: The Building Block

Most people think anything labeled "high protein" is good. But check **how much** you're getting.

For example:

- 2g protein in a ₹60 bar = not worth it
- 15g protein with low sugar = decent
- 20g+ protein with clean ingredients = Jackpot!

Compare per **100g or per serving,** and evaluate if it fits your health goals.

8. Percent Daily Value (%DV): Your Nutrient Compass

This helps you understand **how much of your daily need** is met by one serving.

As a thumb rule:

- **5% or less** = low
- **20% or more** = high

So if a food has **25% sodium,** that's already **one-fourth** of your daily salt intake, in just one serving!

9. Fiber: The Missing Hero

Most packaged foods are fiber-deficient. But **fiber is what slows down sugar absorption,** keeps you full, and helps gut health.

Look for:

- 3g or more fiber per serving = decent
- 5g+ = excellent

High fiber = Low cravings. Period.

10. Health Claims: Don't Fall for the Front

If the front says:

- "100% Natural"
- "Low-Fat"
- "No Added Sugar"
- "Baked, Not Fried"

Just smile... and turn it around.

These terms are **not regulated**. A product can still be full of **chemicals, preservatives**, or **calories**.

You gotta think like a detective. *Label padh, dimaag lagaa, aur health banaa!*

Putting It All Together: Product: Flavored Yogurt

Label Check:

- Serving Size: 100g
- Calories: 180
- Total Sugar: 20g (Added Sugar: 15g)
- Protein: 4g
- Fat: 3g (Saturated: 1.5g)
- Sodium: 120mg

- Fiber: 0g
- Ingredients: Milk, Sugar, Flavoring, Stabilizers, Color 150d

Verdict: Loaded with sugar and artificial stuff. Not healthy, despite the "yogurt" halo.

Quick Look into Calories for your information

Dish	Quantity	Calories (kcal)
Rajma Chawal	250 g	345
Chole Bhature	300 g	450
Dal Makhani	200 g	250
Aloo Paratha (with ghee)	150 g	320
Paneer Butter Masala	200 g	350
Palak Paneer	200 g	300
Chicken Curry	200 g	350
Rogan Josh	200 g	380
Kadhi Pakora	200 g	200
Dosa with Sambar & Chutney	250 g	350
Idli with Sambar	2 idlis + sambar	280
Upma	150 g	250
Pongal (Khara)	200 g	310
Rasam with Rice	250 g	220
Fish Curry	200 g	250
Chicken Chettinad	200 g	370
Pesarattu	150 g	240
Macher Jhol	200 g	280

Shukto	200 g	180
Luchi Alur Dom	2 luchis + curry	400
Ghugni	200 g	230
Momos with chutney	4 pieces	200
Chhena Poda	100 g	300
Dalma	200 g	220
Dhokla	100 g	150
Thepla	70 g	140
Undhiyu	200 g	280
Misal Pav	1 plate	400
Pav Bhaji	1 plate	450
Vada Pav	1 piece	300
Puran Poli	100 g	300
Thukpa	250 ml	250
Bamboo Shoot Pork	200 g	280
Eromba	200 g	180
Jadoh	250 g	350
Fish Tenga	200 g	240
Rice Beer (Apong)	200 ml	150
Smoked Meat with Axone	200 g	300
Samosa	1 piece (~100 g)	308

Gulab Jamun	2 pieces (~100 g)	432
Mysore Pak	100 g	420
Kesari Bath	100 g	300
Rasgulla	2 pieces (~100 g)	300
Sandesh	100 g	250
Shrikhand	100 g	290
Basundi	100 g	320
Sel Roti	1 piece (~100 g)	310
Pitha	1 piece (~100 g)	280
Rice (Brown)	100 g	353.7
Rice (Parboiled)	100 g	351.5
Wheat Flour	100 g	320.2
Ragi	100 g	320.7
Jowar	100 g	334.1
Bajra	100 g	347.9
Bengal Gram Dal	100 g	329.1
Green Gram Dal	100 g	325.7
Red Gram Dal	100 g	330.7
Rajma (Kidney Beans)	100 g	299.2
Carrot	100 g	48

Cauliflower	100 g	30
Spinach	100 g	24.3
Tomato	100 g	21
Potato	100 g	97
Apple	100 g	56
Banana	100 g	95
Mango	100 g	70
Orange	100 g	53
Papaya	100 g	32
Almonds	100 g	602
Cashew Nuts	100 g	582
Peanuts	100 g	567
Milk (Cow's)	100 g	67
Curd	100 g	98
Paneer	100 g	265
Tea (without sugar)	100 g	1
Coffee (without sugar)	100 g	2

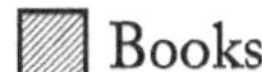 BIBLIOGRAPHY

Books

Baumeister, Roy & Tierney, John. *Willpower: Rediscovering the Greatest Human Strength.* Penguin Books, 2011.

Chopra, Deepak. *Quantum Healing: Exploring the Frontiers of Mind/Body Medicine.* Bantam, 1989.

Clear, James. *Atomic Habits: An Easy & Proven Way to Build Good Habits & Break Bad Ones.* Avery, 2018.

Damodaran, Harish. *India's New Capitalists: Caste, Business, and Industry in a Modern Nation.* Permanent Black, 2008.

Dispenza, Joe. *You Are the Placebo: Making Your Mind Matter.* Hay House, 2014.

Diwekar, Rujuta. *Don't Lose Your Mind, Lose Your Weight.* Westland, 2009.

Duhigg, Charles. *The Power of Habit: Why We Do What We Do in Life and Business.* Random House, 2012.

Dweck, Carol S. *Mindset: The New Psychology of Success.* Ballantine Books, 2006.

Fogg, B.J. *Tiny Habits: The Small Changes That Change Everything.* Houghton Mifflin Harcourt, 2019.

Goggins, David. *Can't Hurt Me.* Lioncrest Publishing, 2018.

Greene, Robert. *The 48 Laws of Power.* Viking Press, 1998.

Holiday, Ryan. *Ego is the Enemy.* Portfolio, 2016.

Holiday, Ryan. *The Obstacle is the Way.* Portfolio, 2014.

Imai, Masaaki. *Kaizen: The Key to Japan's Competitive Success.* McGraw-Hill Education, 1986.

Jain, T.N. *Marwari Wisdom: Traditional Business Practices of India's Greatest Merchants.* HarperBusiness, 2021.

Keller, Gary & Papasan, Jay. *The ONE Thing: The Surprisingly Simple Truth Behind Extraordinary Results*. Bard Press, 2013.

Lieberman, Daniel. *Exercised: Why Something We Never Evolved to Do is Healthy and Rewarding*. Pantheon, 2021.

Manson, Mark. *The Subtle Art of Not Giving a Fck**. Harper, 2016.

Rubin, Gretchen. *Better Than Before: Mastering the Habits of Our Everyday Lives*. Crown Publishing Group, 2015.

Sadhguru. *Inner Engineering: A Yogi's Guide to Joy*. Spiegel & Grau, 2016.

Scott, Jamuna Prasad. *Caste as Social Capital: The Marwaris in India*. Penguin Random House India, 2020.

Sincero, Jen. *You Are a Badass*. Running Press, 2013.

Swartz, Tom. *Many Healthy Adults May Have a Troubling Heart Condition. New York Post*, 2024.

Wayne S. Andersen. *Dr. A's Habits of Health*. Habits of Health Publishing, 2008.

Yogananda, Paramahansa. *Autobiography of a Yogi*. Self-Realization Fellowship, 1946.

▨ Academic Journals, Research & Medical Reports

Baumeister, R.F., & Leary, M.R. (1995). The need to belong: Desire for interpersonal attachments. *Psychological Bulletin*.

Christakis, N.A., & Fowler, J.H. (2007). The Spread of Obesity in a Social Network. *New England Journal of Medicine*.

Deci, E.L., & Ryan, R.M. (2000). The "What" and "Why" of Goal Pursuits. *Psychological Inquiry*.

Fiatarone MA, et al. (1994). Exercise training and nutritional supplementation. *New England Journal of Medicine*.

Frontera WR, et al. (1988). Strength conditioning in older men. *Journal of Applied Physiology*.

Festinger, L. (1954). A Theory of Social Comparison Processes. *Human Relations*.

Goyal, M., Singh, S., et al. (2014). Meditation Programs for Stress. *JAMA Internal Medicine.*

Graybiel, A.M. (2008). Habits, Rituals, and the Brain. *Annual Review of Neuroscience.*

Marlatt, G.A., & Donovan, D.M. (2005). *Relapse Prevention.* Guilford Press.

Norcross, J.C., & Vangarelli, D.J. (1988). The Resolution Solution. *Journal of Substance Abuse.*

Prochaska, J.O., & DiClemente, C.C. (1983). Stages of Self-Change. *Journal of Consulting and Clinical Psychology.*

Prochaska, J.O., & Velicer, W.F. (1997). Transtheoretical Model. *American Journal of Health Promotion.*

Roubenoff, R. (2000). Sarcopenia in Elderly. *European Journal of Clinical Nutrition.*

Sallis, J.F., & Owen, N. (1999). *Physical Activity and Behavioral Medicine.* SAGE Publications.

Selye, H. (1950). The General Adaptation Syndrome. *British Medical Journal.*

Quinn, T. J., & Coons, B. A. (2011). The talk test and its relationship with the ventilatory and lactate thresholds. Journal of Sports Sciences, 29(11), 1175-1182. NASM Blog. (2020).

Recalde, P. T., Foster, C., & Porcari, J. P. (2020). The validity of the talk test for prescribing and monitoring exercise intensity. International Journal of Sports Physiology and Performance, 15(8), 1192-1198.

▩ Government, Institutes & Online Reports

Food Safety and Standards Authority of India (FSSAI). *Consumer Guidance Reports.*

Harvard Medical School. *Reports on Mindfulness, Sleep, and Nutrition,* various years.

Harvard Business Review. *Kaizen & Behavioral Psychology Articles,* various.

Indian Ministry of Health and Family Welfare. *NCD and Health Surveillance Reports.*

National Council for Biotechnology Information (NCBI). *Muscle metabolism studies.*

National Programme for Health Care of the Elderly (India). *Elder Care Reports.*

NSCA (National Strength and Conditioning Association). *Trainer Resources and Research.*

Pew Research Center. *Millennials, Gen Z & Social Media Studies.*

Statista. (2023). *Global Social Media & Lifestyle Data.*

University of Scranton. (2014). *Why 92% of Resolutions Fail. Journal of Clinical Psychology.*

WHO (World Health Organization). (2022). *Depression and Common Mental Disorders.*

Krstev Barać, Sandra. *Nutrition, Exercise and Optimal Body Composition*

ABOUT THE AUTHOR

Akash Jaiswal is not just a name; he is a living, breathing example of resilience, reinvention, and relentless self-belief. Akash Jaiswal is a Semiconductor Industry Professional, with a master's degree from NIT Kurukshetra. But beyond the labs and logic gates lies a story of extraordinary transformation.

Once weighing over 90 kilograms, Akash embarked on a powerful journey of self-discipline, shedding fat, gaining muscle, and ultimately securing 3rd prize in a district-level bodybuilding championship. He has also completed more than three marathons, each one a milestone in his commitment to mental and physical resilience.

After his debut book, *I Too Can Create*, which inspired readers to tap into their creative potential to Social Media, Akash penned *Zero to Everyone*, a guide for startups looking to go from obscurity to market dominance. His third and most personal book, *Zip It Up*, takes a bold step into the world of health, mindset, and transformation. It's not just a book; it's a mirror for anyone who has ever felt stuck, overweight, or unworthy, and a roadmap to getting their power back.

Through his story, Akash hopes to show that change is possible, not just for the few, but for anyone willing to commit, struggle, and rise again.